# Process Work in Person-Centred Therapy

*Also by Richard Worsley*

HUMAN FREEDOM AND THE LOGIC OF EVIL: PROLEGOMENON TO A CHRISTIAN THEOLOGY OF EVIL

THE INTEGRATIVE PRIMER: AN INTRODUCTION TO INTEGRATIVE COUNSELLING WITH A PERSON-CENTRED FOUNDATION

*Co-edited with Professor Stephen Joseph*

PERSON-CENTRED PSYCHOPATHOLOGY: A POSITIVE PSYCHOLOGY OF MENTAL HEALTH

PERSON-CENTRED PRACTICE: CASE STUDIES IN POSITIVE PSYCHOLOGY

# Process Work in Person-Centred Therapy

## 2nd Edition

Richard Worsley

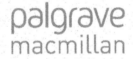

palgrave
macmillan

First published 2001
Second edition published 2009 by
PALGRAVE MACMILLAN

Palgrave Macmillan in the UK is an imprint of Macmillan Publishers Limited,
registered in England, company number 785998, of Houndmills, Basingstoke,
Hampshire RG21 6XS.

Palgrave Macmillan in the US is a division of St Martin's Press LLC,
175 Fifth Avenue, New York, NY 10010.

Palgrave Macmillan is the global academic imprint of the above companies
and has companies and representatives throughout the world.

Palgrave® and Macmillan® are registered trademarks in the United States,
the United Kingdom, Europe and other countries.

ISBN 978-0-230-21315-9     ISBN 978-1-137-28586-7 (eBook)
DOI 10.1007/978-1-137-28586-7

This book is printed on paper suitable for recycling and made from fully
managed and sustained forest sources. Logging, pulping and manufacturing
processes are expected to conform to the environmental regulations of the
country of origin.

A catalogue record for this book is available from the British Library.

A catalog record for this book is available from the Library of Congress.

10   9   8   7   6   5   4   3   2   1
18   17   16   15   14   13   12   11   10   09

*To Jack and Kathleen who gave me a secure base
and love without question.*

*To Margaret and Leonard who became a second family
without parallel.*

*To Chris, Susan, Rachel and Jonathan whose
love and scepticism sustain me.*

*To the congregations of the parishes where I have ministered,
who taught me of the love that is fulsome. It is the basis of
person-centred therapy too.*

# Contents

# Preface

Being a person-centred therapist is to make a conscious and rational commitment to trusting the potential of the client in the face of all that life can bring. I work with people because I believe that they can, in my company as well as by themselves, draw near to that process of living that Carl Rogers calls 'fully functioning' (Rogers, 1957b). To be fully functioning is not to have reached some ultimate goal. Rather, it is to be in a fluent process of becoming, of living in growing awareness of one's thinking, feeling and bodily sensation; to be more alive in the present; to be open to experience of self and others; to be fulfilling one's needs and therefore to be able to live for others as well. This is just some of what it is to live authentically.

I see humans as trustworthy, not because of some philosophical generalization, but because, in intuiting their resources, I choose to live with faith in them and notice that, when I do this, they locate their potential, by and large. I have learned from clients, from trusting in natural process, that those issues which bring clients to therapy are clearly not normally illnesses to be cured, but ways in which the natural organism expresses its need. I trust people to find better, more functional ways of expressing this need, if I can provide them with the conditions to do this.

As I have grown in experience as a therapist, not least through teaching therapy for seven years, and now as someone who sees about 20 clients a week for most weeks of my year, I have come to recognize that there is a need to think radically about how I interact with clients and how I use both person-centred and other phenomenological and existential theories to inform my practice. This book is the fruit of being puzzled, curious and, I hope, creative in the context of years of teaching and doing therapy. It is therefore an invitation to the reader to embark on a similar journey. It will not be *my* journey, even if it is dialogue with what I have written. It will be yours.

To be person-centred is to resist the constriction of life's many *oughts*. It is to find freedom. As therapists develop, the more creative among us will recognize their need to find a freedom to practice as themselves (Tudor and Worrall, 2004). The commitment to grow into such freedom is at the centre of this book.

# Acknowledgements

This book is the product of the work and dedication of many minds. In particular, I want to thank:

- my colleagues who have thought through the implications of being person-centred with me in my teaching at City College, Coventry: Anne Booth, Maggie Fuller, Sandra Grainger, Jim Murphy, Janet McNaught, Tracey Sanders, Janette Torrance, John White;
- my colleagues who have shared with me the day to day work of counseling staff and students at the University of Warwick: Peter Byrd, Shirley Crookes, Hanya Czepkowski, Maureen Haynes, Pualine McManus, Anthea Pablow, Samantha Tarren, Linda Watkinson;
- those who have been my students, my clients and my supervisees, who although invisible have been the bedrock of my practice and learning;
- those who have shared with me in supervision, and have challenged me from many perspectives: Nic Blackwell, Fran Bradley, David Charles-Edwards, Moira Fryer, Chris Rose;
- to Pete Sanders and Maggie Taylor-Sanders for their wisdom, friendship and commitment, and to Pete for reading the first edition of this book critically for me;
- to those who have read drafts of this book and given invaluable feedback: Nick Baker, Dave Mearns, Pete Sanders, Brain Thorne, Janette Torrance;
- to the staff of Palgrave, and amongst them Frances Arnold and Alison Dixon, but in particular to Catherine Gray for her wisdom and critical insight in helping me steer through the second edition of this book.

# Who Is This Book For?

The first edition of the book was published in 2002. I am grateful for the feedback and the affirmation I have had, that this is a text that is useful, and that, once picked up, it is treated with affection. It is intended for:

- teachers of counselling and counselling skills;
- person-centred and humanistic practitioners, particularly those with an interest in their own freedom to practice;
- supervisors of person-centred or humanistic counsellors;
- people working for Masters degrees in counselling or counselling psychology or Masters or Doctorates in clinical psychology;
- students beginning the second year of counselling diploma courses, in particular person-centred or humanistic diplomas, who want to explore their own ways of being person-centred;
- others who want something of a flavour of practice issues current within the person-centred approach.

I have come to appreciate that others from beyond the person-centred fold have benefitted from the book. The book addresses how clients construct process internally, and that is important theory for all therapists, of whatever orientation. It invites us to consider how we might challenge and support clients in their existential quest for authenticity. In this it offers a view of what Dave Mearns and Mick Cooper (2005) have come to refer to as *relational depth*. It resonates with counsellors who are either committed to, or just plain puzzled about, both the existential and the spiritual in life. Beyond the discipline of therapy, the book was warmly received, for instance, by a colleague who is a specialist in management development in industrial and educational settings.

## Process Work – Introducing the Question

The logical starting point of the book is to note that the person-centred family is a vexatious and divided one, at times. The main division is between those who take a classical, client-centred approach, sometimes referred to as a purist or literalist approach, and those who are experientialist or process-orientated. (These terms and others will be explained later in the book.) The aim of

this book is twofold. First it suggests that this toxic dichotomy is unnecessary, in that there are ways in which the insights of both camps can be
honoured, but with moderation. However, if it were merely a seeking for a
middle way, that could be insipid! Rather the book challenges the reader to
think hard about very familiar concepts, like the necessity and sufficiency of
the core conditions, and then to consider radically what is coherent in her
own practice. Only through hard thought and analysis will we find freedom to
practice.

   The basic argument of this book is that it is both possible and desirable to
address oneself towards the client's process, and that, as therapists and clients,
we can address ourselves towards our own process. Indeed it is impossible
to avoid doing these things. However, unlike some of the experiential psychotherapists (for instance, Greenberg *et al.*, 1993), this can be done in such
a way as to respect both the client's own actualizing tendency; the principle
of non-directiveness; and the six conditions of therapy (Rogers, 1957a). In
order to address the client's process, it is important to remember its basis in
the phenomenological and existential principles which underlie all humanistic
therapies. As part of this argument, I illustrate how other humanistic therapies – in particular, Transactional Analysis and Gestalt therapy – can inform
our understanding of client process. When I first wrote these chapters, in
2000–2002, my sole intention was to demonstrate the usefulness of other,
congruent theories to develop our understanding of client process. However,
it turns out that I had set a hare running that others have chased – that of
*integration*. Two years after the publication of the first edition of this book,
I contributed a chapter (Worsley, 2004) to Pete Sanders' (2004) *Tribes of the
Person-Centered Nation*. I argued there that theoretical material from many
approaches could be integrated into person-centred work such that the latter
maintained its essential integrity. This has had much effect upon its readers, it
seems. A number of people have told me that they derived from this chapter
permission to think more freely, less constrainedly, about how they practised.
Freedom to practice is crucial. However, it cannot be irresponsible freedom.
We must always be able to give an account of why we think that what we do
is coherent. *Freedom to practice is rooted in an exploration of all that might
be possible together with a properly critical adherence to the core principles of the
approach.*

## Chapter by Chapter

Chapter 1 is an introduction to the key terms and ideas of process work,
rooted in the case of Henry. Chapter 2 of this book will elaborate upon this
first view of process work, against a background of the controversy between
those who follow a literal and experiential approach, suggesting that there is

a rationale for addressing the client's process without ceasing to be person-centred. Chapter 3 locates it in terms of Carl Rogers' work on process in psychotherapy.

Part II of the book examines the consequences of understanding person-centred therapy as applied phenomenology. Chapter 4 introduces the concept of phenomenology. Chapter 5 explores narrative and metaphor as aspects of the client's phenomenology. Chapters 6 and 7 argue that the client's phenomenology can be experienced through the language and concepts of other phenomenologically orientated therapies such as Transactional Analysis and Gestalt therapy. Chapter 8 examines the consequences of a phenomenological perspective upon the therapist in terms of the freedom to practise as oneself.

In Part III, the case for an existential perspective is developed. While almost all person-centred practitioners will see the discipline as rooted in phenomenology, the claim that it is rooted also in existentialism is more controversial, not least because the person-centred movement finds its origin in American optimism, whereas existentialism is darkly European. In Chapter 9, the case for the existential perspective begins with the work of Martin Buber, and his consideration of the nature of relating. This is then opened up in Chapter 10 in more general philosophical terms, looking to examine what life commitments the person-centred practitioner needs to acknowledge, and how this might impact upon client work. Chapter 11 moves beyond the existential to current debates in the spirituality of counselling, in order to countenance the possibility that the material often called spiritual is also part of the client's process.

Part IV uses in Chapter 12 concepts from person-centred psychopathology to illuminate normal-range process work with clients. Chapter 13 offers a paradigm for addressing process from the work of Les Greenberg, Laura Rice and Robert Elliott, followed by a case study of Hilary as a brief example of working with process, and with this paradigm in particular. The final chapter draws together the many threads of the book at the level of practice.

## The Changing and Growing World of Person-Centred Therapy

The need for a second edition of this book springs almost wholly from the fact that the theory and practice of person-centred therapy are changing and growing fast. The question of *integration* within person-centred therapy is one that is emerging from the woodwork. I say this as a teacher of counselling. I used to watch a small number of students of counselling experiencing a crisis of faith in the person-centred belief system. I can recall how beguiling Gestalt can be. Now we can really intervene and *do* something for the client. (Of course, good

Gestaltists have got beyond this illusion!) It has become increasingly important that the possibility of integration should be offered, so that it does not
happen anyway in an irresponsible and even eclectic manner. In the long term,
therapies of all orientations will need to converge. I felt a real sorrow that
this book has no adequate room for considering object relations theory and
therapy in particular. This has been an important part of my own growth.

For Carl Rogers, the self seemed to be best conceptualized as a unitary system in which internal communication is fluent and congruent with
the empirical world. Such diverse streams of thought as psychodynamic theory, neuro-science and postmodern philosophy have brought this unitary self
deeply and rightly into question. Recently, there has been much fruitful work
on the notion that the *self is multiple* (Rowan, 1990; Cooper, 1999, 2005;
Mearns and Thorne, 2000). This has direct relevance to client process. Once
we can picture the client as the gestalt of a multiplicity of configurations, we
have new ways of thinking and speaking about clients, and of working with
them.

Perhaps the most important new work that is engaging an increasing
number of practitioners concerns person-centred *psychopathology* (Joseph and
Worsley, 2005; Worsley and Joseph, 2007). One stereotype of person-centred
therapy has been that it is short on theory and only useable with the 'worried well'. The work of Garry Prouty and of Margaret Warner with people
with schizophrenia, in the United States, and of Dion van Werde and Marlis
Pörtner in Europe has been fundamental in recasting person-centred therapy
as a theory which can describe accurately severe dysfunction, and a therapy
that can address it (Prouty, van Werde and Pörtner, 2002; Warner, 2002,
2007). Alongside this new approach to severely disturbed clients has come
an awareness of the existential meaning of depression in particular (Cooper,
2003; Worsley, 2007). In turn this speaks to those psychologists who are
paying renewed attention to positive psychology, which is not merely the psychology of well-being, of happiness, but a deeper consideration of the role of
affirmation of the client's process even when it is painful (Linley and Joseph,
2004). The concerns of this book are being echoed as green shoots in clinical
psychology by people who may never have come across Carl Rogers!

Alongside Mearns and Cooper's (2005) consideration of relational depth
sits the work of the Austrian academic and therapist, Peter Schmid. He strives
to conceptualize therapy in terms of *encounter*, and of the ethical demands of
each person upon the other within that encounter (Schmid, 1998, 2006). It
seems to me that he has tapped into important new concepts but also new
resources. Not least amongst these is the work of the French philosopher,
Emmanuel Levinas. I have argued elsewhere (Worsley, 2006) for his importance. Here I incorporate some of his insights into my consideration of both
existentialism and spirituality.

Finally, I want to argue for the spiritual – with all of its slipperiness of
meaning – as an aspect of the client's process which makes quite specific and

stretching demands upon the therapist. Much has been written since 2002 about the *spirituality of counselling*. As a subject it is still in its infancy. We can wait with bated breath for the emergence of new perspectives.

Person-Centred therapy is alive and well in many parts of the world, to judge by the rate of change and growth we are seeing.

## Language and Confidentiality

All case material in this book is fictional, in that I have taken themes from my own experience as a therapist, tried consciously to associate these with particular clients so as to bracket out references which might be identified with the client, and then developed a narrative which is strictly separate from any real-life client whom I can recall – a psychologically real fiction. Where possible, I have sought the permission of clients to use themes and motifs from their work, even though these are not identifiable with the individuals concerned. I am grateful to my clients who have given me consent to use their themes and metaphors for the benefit of others.

There are three exceptions to this. My letter to 'Alistair' in Chapter 5 is a real document used with the client, and used here with his informed consent, although with details changed to preserve anonymity. The aim of the document was research for this book; I do not in the normal course of therapy write to my clients in this way! Chapters 1 and 13 were read and amended by 'Henry' and 'Hilary' respectively, in first draft. I am grateful that they were willing to allow me to use their material.

I aim throughout to speak in a gender-inclusive fashion. I habitually refer to the reader, the client and others in the feminine, occasionally in the masculine, so as to avoid contorted usage, but hope that it will be understood that all are included.

I also use the word 'Rogerian' on a number of occasions. I note that others use it in a way I find contentious, as in the phrase 'Rogerian person-centred'. This would imply that there is a characteristic way of being person-centred that belongs to Rogers, and that other ways of being person-centred do not. A number of essays in Farber *et al.* (1996) bring this into question. The year before his death, and after a demonstration session, a student pointed out that Rogers' use of questions was not what the student's lecturer had said was right. Carl Rogers reflected for a few moments and commented that one of the privileges he had was that he did not need to be Rogerian! I use the word 'Rogerian' in a strictly analytic sense, meaning: of or pertaining to the work, writing or thought of Carl Rogers.

# 1

# Process and Listening

## A Case Study in Process

> Ah! A chocolate biscuit! How nice! I shouldn't.... But I am going to!

I do not know how many times in a year I play out this strange little verbal ritual about being offered a chocolate biscuit. Perhaps my colleagues at work are tired of it. Yet, counsellors do find biscuits a good way to alleviate tiredness. Behind the words over the biscuit lie quite complicated processes, I suspect. Firstly, because it is a ritual, it is also a game. I expect others not to take me too seriously. Secondly, I suspect this means that I am quite serious about what is going on. It starts with my body and my nose and my eyes. It centres on the biscuit, of course. I want it. I mean I *really* want it. Nothing appeals like temptation. I then act out an inner conflict, but fairly light-heartedly. The conflict is between my need to enjoy something sweet and my need to watch my diet. However, I suspect other things are going on. I seem to need to 'amuse' others with this conflict. I notice I feel far from comfortable acknowledging this to myself. Perhaps they would like me to stop doing it. But I won't! I am proud of being determined, but my Dad called it being stubborn. Being determined (or stubborn) helps me sometimes to give containment to fragile clients. Perhaps I use it to keep the diet going, but in a way that isn't too strict. Or perhaps it is all about a bit of irritating exhibitionism. The point is, even I cannot be sure. And, if I can't be sure about my process, you certainly couldn't, at least not without a lot of shared exploration.

Even eating a chocolate biscuit seems to involve a lot of interesting process. Some of this I can be quite sure about. Other aspects of it make me feel uncertain, and even rather chary of exploring it. This is a book about process in counselling. Process is not easy to 'get'. When I use the word 'get', I imply that process, as a concept and as a practical understanding, cannot be defined adequately. It has to be intuited. That is because it is something under the surface of all communication, hovering between what we are keenly aware of and that which is beyond our immediate awareness. A definition provides

1

only conceptual understanding, a known meaning. Intuition provides a grasp of a complex phenomenon at a gut level. When I intuit, I am not bound by words and intellect. I am freed to *experience* meaning within me. If I understand a definition, the best I will say is, I know about that now. If I intuit something, I will say, I recognize that, because I have tasted it; but with more experience I will recognize it more fully. This book aims to provide an intuitive recognition of process, and then to help the reader consider how this act of recognizing might legitimately nourish the art of person-centred therapy.

In this chapter, I set out the case of Henry, as a way to think through and recognize process in both client and therapist. This description of work with Henry does not portray process as simple, straightforward. If I tried to make it simpler, I would deceive you. The process of the client, that of the therapist and even that of the therapist's supervisor interweave. While the background is important, I focus near the end of the account upon one particular interaction, over two weeks, between Henry and me. Because thinking about process is never simple, I offer, at the beginning of the next chapter, another type of account of process, as well.

### Case 1.1   Henry

Henry had arrived at my front door looking wet and bedraggled. The rain had come down in torrents at the last minute, and he had no raincoat with him. His umbrella had not protected his suit. He had come direct from his office. His jacket was shiny at the elbows and his trousers needed a press. He looked exhausted. Over the next two and a half years, we worked together, albeit with one break of four months, after the birth of Henry's first child. However, I could not forget that first impression of him as so tired and not a little bedraggled. While he was mainly smart and brisk, at least on the surface, what I first saw remained with me as an image of his discouragement in life.

Henry was aged 34, and was a slight figure of a man. He struggled to eat enough. Some days he looked slim, and on other days he looked drawn. He worked as an executive with a small, scientific instruments firm. He explained at that first meeting that executive was a strange word. It made him seem better at what he did that he thought he was. Henry's fragile surface was well-enough groomed. His dark hair and olive skin at times looked positively handsome. Yet, beneath this veneer was a well of depression that felt to me to be of huge depth, a bottomless pit.

Henry's swarthy looks witnessed to a fascinating family background. His father, older than his mother by some 15 years, had been part of a trade delegation to Sri Lanka. There, he met and married Henry's mother, a Sinhalese Buddhist. She struggled to survive being uprooted from her family and culture to live a very 'English' life – at least on the surface. Henry's father had married late, and rather in desperation, I suspect. There seemed little love lost between Henry's parents. Henry's father was cold and rejecting of Henry, a replica indeed of his own father. The mother was lost in an unfamiliar country and felt that she could not cope. She seems to have moved between feeling depressed and being aggressive towards Henry in her attempts to survive. When Henry was nine years old his father left his mother.

I have often noted that when parents split up, children, especially those before the age of puberty, are left with a terrible dilemma. Who has left whom, and why? Adult logic sees an adult relationship failing. The child, often haunted with incomplete memories of distress, conflict and loneliness, feels that it is he, the child, who has been deserted. There is a primitive process, another version of logic if you will, in operation. The child has to make sense of this from his own resources, and these can be quite thin. Some days I would see glimpses of this confused and angry child trying desperately to make sense of it all appearing beneath Henry's professional veneer. Anger with the father seemed pointless. Henry's feelings seemed pointless. They could rot, as far as others were concerned. If the pain was so great, then the conclusion was inevitable for any child. Such punishment was definitive. It was Henry's fault. He was hateful. He had contaminated his parents' marriage, and it had broken like an abused toy. Henry's self-condemnation knew no bounds.

Henry was intellectually most able. Bullied at school with few friends, he had little to distract him from his studies. He opted to go to Manchester Business School. I reflected that he seemed to be following in his lost father's footsteps. However, his time there had been traumatic. He had suffered his first major bout of depression, and had to take a year out to complete his studies, but more to the point had become saturated with a desire for a string of sexual liaisons which were as personally vacuous for him as they were torrid. At least one of his girlfriends, and the one boy he experimented in sleeping with, managed to exploit him financially to the tune of several hundreds of pounds. Until his late twenties, Henry vacillated between intense loneliness and sexual encounters which spoke deeply of his need for genuine love and approval. I could applaud what he was seeking, but he could not. It was only another sign of his weakness, and a proof that what he had worked out about himself more than a decade ago must be true.

Five years before coming to see me he had met and then married Jennifer. I never met her, but she seemed by all accounts a genuinely loving person, who, although more pedestrian than Henry, was a source for him of stability. He also admired her. Marriage had not been easy. After 18 months, Jenny miscarried their first child. They were both devastated. Instead of giving support, Henry felt again the call of the wild! Other women, the old pattern, became a huge part of his life. Was it just gratification or was it more: the illusory or even real means of exiting into a new life? At about the time of his marriage to Jenny, Henry had returned, somewhat to his astonishment, to his mother's Buddhist faith and practice. He found some comfort in meditation. The image of letting go of attachment and of seeking some form of perfection strengthened him, but at other time intimidated and haunted him.

We spent many a long week working upon Henry's feelings of worthlessness and of hopeless depression. Looking back, I struggle to remember the full course of the therapy, but was aware of the endless circling around Henry's conviction that he deserved all he got, and was somehow perverse in his badness. Even in the first group of sessions, lasting some 20 months, I could alternate between deep affection for Henry and a scarce muted fury at his ability to believe himself of no worth and yet to insist against every fibre in my body that he just *knew* he was rotten to the core.

I came to think of this as cognitive stuckness. I even contemplated a referral for cognitive–behavioural therapy. (Let someone else try to unstick this!) One day, however, Henry gave me a glimpse of another world. He suddenly looked at me and asked, The death of our baby. Tell me it's my *karma* and not Jenny's. In spite of a degree in theology, I found myself disorientated. Surely Buddhism came into being to get rid of the problem of *karma* as it had been in Hinduism. Some quick reading between sessions re-orientated me. For Henry, as for his mother, *karma* is one of a number of forces in our life. It is the weight of sin from past lives, if you will. Yet, Buddhism offers hope that *karma* is not malign. While the West deals in forgiveness, religiously, Buddhism finds hope in the fact that the bad can be wiped out, just like the repayment of a debt. The debt, the sin, is earned, deserved.

I wondered how I would respond in the next session. However, the chance never came. Like so much that is fascinating in counselling, the question of *karma* disappeared – and just when I had found out something about it! However, I could see the Buddhist doctrine as a fascinating aspect of Henry's awareness. The misdeeds in past lives looked very much like his pondering in childhood what must have been his twistedness that caused his father to leave and his mother to be perpetually angry. Yet, Henry's ability to meditate upon his own pain, together with the doctrine of *karma*, offered him a way out of the absoluteness of his self-condemnation. Even more, he wanted to protect Jenny from karmic vindication. He could seek to preserve that which he loved.

Bit by bit, the depression lifted. At about this time, Henry left therapy because of the birth of their new child. Expense and exhaustion took away from him the resources to pay much attention to himself.

Four months later, he returned. I had not expected that. I was glad to see him, but thrown by his state of mind. He was down. He was flat. He hated himself. Strangely, he said that he did not exactly feel depressed. He just felt awful. The shield of depression had lifted. He had moved from helplessness and lack of emotional intensity to a simple state of pain. He was in the depths of despair, but in such a way that the experience seemed to have a strange purity to it. I could feel within me some of my old irritation with Henry's implacable, grinding self-condemnation. Neither Jenny's everyday love nor the gift of a child alleviated this. In other circumstances I would have needed to work my way towards being able to be immersed in this dark field for month after month.

However, there was an external problem. My partner's job was taking us away from the area. This was the end of my private practice, and I had this to grieve too. One of my supervisees was working her way through her anger with me for going only eight months after taking her on. So, Henry too was going to be short-term! Perhaps all I had to offer him was the ending. I encouraged him to see an ending in the very short term indeed. I was desperate that he just got to grips with what we had learned before. In short, the ending made me want to rescue him by getting the cognitive stuff into place, and the need to do so made me press even harder than circumstances required for an ending. We agreed – or at least I specified – an ending for mid-November. I was moving in the New Year.

Henry commented resentfully that all that counselling seemed to have done for him was to make him feel the pain of despair more acutely.

We resumed our second set of sessions with about five sessions to go, although eleven would have been possible, practically. While the precise content of each session seems to me less that relevant now,

I was increasingly aware that Henry had come back feeling utterly stuck in his pain. The depression seemed to have moved away, and what remained felt raw. In the first set of sessions, Henry had begun to develop some sense of how his present and his past connected. Some clients can see the past as a true explanation of the present in a way that is really useful to them. (See, for instance, Hilary in Chapter 13.) Others seem not to need to visit the past at all. Acceptance and empathy in the present connects for them. For Henry, the past seemed a useful but alien territory. Yes, he could grant that his childhood had been painful, even that it had distorted his perception of himself. But only rarely did this seem to help him locate a felt-shift in his emotions.

Over some three sessions, I noticed that I was working very hard, and desperately wanted Henry to forge connections with his past. Perhaps I expected Henry to have a rational relationship with himself, in spite of what I knew about emotions. Since he knew the origin of his sense of self-rejection he should surely forgive himself! At worst, I became acutely aware of Henry, under pressure from me, meeting time and again those parts of himself he detested, and when invited to consider what they meant, would say, Don't know! Of course, he wasn't wrong. But I could not get why I could feel so irritated about this. Sometimes it can take hard thinking and too much time for a stuck therapist to get what is going on – the process.

What finally dawned upon me was that there was no gap – literally no time gap – between what I said and Henry's 'Don't know'! He did not stop to think. And my irritation? Henry felt like a sullen teenager. He wasn't trying. He wasn't on my side. Eventually I turned that round. Maybe I wasn't on his side either. Something had to shift. It was a shift inside me that mattered. Only then could Henry and I shift together.

The next session, I told Henry that I was aware that I wanted to get the ending done and help him to survive without me, to solve how he was for himself. I told him that I thought this would no longer do, and that he could have the seven or so sessions that remained to him; that he would need to construct his own ending with me; that I was going to get off his case and stop trying to be at all helpful. Finally I added that it really was his job, and that how he did with it was up to him. I was a companion on that journey but no more. (I winced. Did that sound harsh? It was not meant to.) Henry took on board what I said. Considering what a hole I had dug for myself over three sessions, I thought he did this very graciously. I might have been rather more pissed off with me.

The next session, I could feel myself settling down into my chair. I felt warm and comfortable and, well, just less responsible. I cannot recall what Henry talked about at first. I do remember how much I enjoyed listening to him. Then, about half way through the session, Henry looked at me and said, I guess when I am under this sort of pressure I regress to a default position, and that is my teenage years. I simply echoed his words: When life hurts, it's as if you become a sullen teenager again. That is such a simple response, but I wanted to emblazon it across the sky. Why? I guess from that point onwards I thought that a real shift was happening. What is the process? To understand process, we must begin with the very bedrock of person-centred therapy.

## The Bedrock of Person-Centred Therapy

The starting point of all person-centred therapy must be the therapist's trust in the client's *actualizing tendency*, the natural, organismic potential of the client to seek to lower psychological incongruence, the tension between the outer manifestations of the client's life and his view of himself (Rogers, 1963). The therapist is committed in all that she does to allow this natural process to take place. In all forms of counselling it is ethically crucial that the client is accorded respect and autonomy, the right to make his own decisions. However, in person-centred therapy, autonomy is also about the very process of change. In short, we do not use tool-like actions and activities to do things to the client. The language of treatment sits ill with the person-centred approach. Therapist and client are engaged in shared process.

It is often said that the therapist does not take an expert stance. There is much truth in this. Expertise can alienate the therapist from the world of the client as the client knows it (Sanders, 2007a). However, to renounce all expertise is a gross oversimplification. David Rennie (1998) argues that the therapist is an expert on the client's process, but the client is the expert on his lived experience. This too is very rigid. Perhaps, in meeting, each person brings expertise of sorts. Only the client can know at first hand his experience. The therapist finally has little choice but to trust this. However, she is free to challenge what she hears. All good challenge clarifies, without unduly distorting the power dynamics of a sound relationship.

Carl Rogers (1951, 1957a, 1959) asked what it was that made non-directive therapy – as he termed person-centred therapy in its earliest days – effective. He formulated the six conditions of therapy. (See Chapter 3.) This summary of a structure and a quality of relating is often abbreviated to the three core conditions of empathy, congruence and unconditional positive regard. I will argue in Chapter 3 that process work need not depart from the six conditions of therapy. The core conditions set out a *quality* of relating. However, as such, they do not tell the therapist what to do. She has to decide how to implement these conditions. There are perhaps as many ways of doing this as there are competent therapists. There is room for responsible experiment, a growing into the freedom to practice.

If the bedrock of person-centred therapy is the according of a quality of relationship which allows the client's actualizing tendency elbow room to find its own wisdom, its own path, then consequently there is no one right way of acting. There are no set pieces. There is no correct set of verbal activities in which to indulge. It has been said, for instance, that the therapist must track the client, following him in all he says. (This is adhering to the client's frame of reference.) This is naturally a pretty useful thing to do for much of the time. Yet, Maria Villas-Boas Bowen (1996) has shown that Carl Rogers spoke from his own frame of reference in his recorded sessions sometimes as little as 4 per cent of the time, but sometimes as much as 22 per cent of the time. There must be an element of clinical judgement here. (How strong is the client's sense of self?) But Villas-Boas Bowen hypothesizes that Rogers began to speak more from his own frame of reference as he matured because he came to be more trusting of the client in his latter years.

Within the 'nation' of person-centred and experiential therapies (Sanders, 2004), there is much variety and not a little dispute. Some experiential work does seem to be directive. Peter Sanders, in his address to the Chicago Conference of the World Association for Person-Centered and Experiential Psychotherapy and Counseling, 2000, offered a clear, democratic and non-judgemental way of thinking about the differences between practices and practitioners. Again I will examine this in Chapter 2.

## The Phenomenological Stance

Part of the bedrock of person-centred therapy is rooted in phenomenology, a philosophical theory about the nature of human experiencing. This is explored in some depth in Chapter 4. At heart, phenomenology says that when we experience something, it is not the object itself we experience and report. That is always and ever elusively 'out there'. Reported experience is interpreted, put together by us in our own characteristic way. Thus, when I say that I feel angry, I may mean something very different from what you mean when you use the identical words. This analysis of human experiencing has two consequences for therapists.

Firstly, if my experience is unique to me, because I put it together in my own fashion, then the only way you can understand me is to explore with me at some length and depth what I actually experience. This means listening carefully, imagining within limits (empathy), using your own not-knowing creatively, challenging what I say, and finally having to trust my experience as my own. (The last two of these are in real tension, because there is such a thing as self-deception.)

Secondly, the founder of phenomenology, the German philosopher Edmund Husserl, proposed in his 1931 book *Ideas* that all experience has two elements to it. He labeled these with the Greek words *noema* and *noesis*. These are not easy words to define. However, they are very important words to wrestle with. They are sometimes described as the What and the How of experiencing, sometimes as the content and the texture of our experiencing. The *noema* points to the 'object' of what we experience. If I look at a tree, and recognize it as a tree, then the *noema* of my experience is its 'treeness'.

It is the *noesis* that matter here. The *noesis* of my experience of a tree might be in its greenness, its sense of natural beauty, its evoking in me childhood memories of climbing and of freedom and so forth. The word 'texture' is useful but in the end is too passive. I put together each experience actively. When I look at a tree, then I can speak about the way I put together my experience of a tree.

To return to anger, the sheer variety of experiences that this word subsumes is down to the fact that different people put together their anger in vastly different ways. The way I assemble my experiences is deeply connected with their meaning for me. Existentialism is one way of thinking of humans as meaning-generating animals. We generate meaning from the way we assemble our experiencing (Gendlin, 1997). This is why this book has to take seriously the existential. Therapists do not just meet the clients' experiences, but are involved at all times in the client's generation of meaning and thus in their own life-meanings as well.

What then is process work? Each chapter will seem to give a slightly different cut through this question. Yet, each will add richness and detail to the basic answer: process work is the commitment by the therapist to pay full attention to, and interact with, the *noesis* of the client's experiencing. How we put experience together is as important as what we report that experience to be. Carl Rogers' descriptions of incongruence are all concerned with the *noesis* of experience. It is at the heart of person-centre therapy.

The emphasis of this book suggests that some classical, client-centred therapists understate the importance of process. For those for whom this is not the case, I am glad. Some experiential therapists overstate the role of direction and prescription in therapy. For those for whom this is not the case, I rejoice.

## Process Work in Action

Henry is now in the process of change. I will never know the end of this. My move has robbed me of this, but perhaps we never know the end of things for our clients, because therapy is only a small part of the journey of life. Henry is in change. Henry is in process. How can I understand this process, looking back?

Where did process change?

For me, the answer is surprising but most important. At one level, change happened within my supervisor. She is a woman of great experience and wisdom, who has learned over the years to trust her own processing. She had supported me in my perceived need to ensure a 'positive' – swift? – ending with Henry. When I got stuck with Henry's implacable 'Don't Know!' she recalled a client of hers. She had made a swift ending after a very long piece of work. She recalled her subsequent regret. This process, this act of memory, was perhaps the crucial change. Within her, first of all, the *noesis*, the meaning, feel and texture of ending had shifted. I was able to recycle this as permission to question radically where I was with Henry.

Intersecting with this was another change in process. Before returning to me, Henry had stopped processing his life-dilemmas as depression. The blanket of depression had lifted. Feelings were no longer damped down. Clients often feel worse before they feel better. Henry resented this, and perhaps resented me for achieving this with him. Now we were faced with raw pain.

As mature practitioners, we still rely upon the affirmation that goes with things going well. It is good up to a point. Beyond that point the need to be successful in a therapist is toxic. I now see that under the pressure of the move I simply resented having to re-engage with Henry's pain. So solid, and dense! So raw! I do not say that with self-blame. Rather I regret missing something about the quality of my irritation with Henry. In the first set of sessions I could stand back and see my irritation as a natural reaction against his profound stuckness. I sort of sided with his constructive self in bringing into impatient question the certainty he felt of his own perverseness. What I missed with my irritation with his pain when he returned was that I was unable to remain with not just his pain but also my irritation. I simply wanted him to have learned enough, cognitively, to fix himself. One does not have to be into very advanced theory to spot that this will not do.

At times we have to be 'bad' therapists, missing the obvious, to pick up the full process of our interactions. I needed to get in some way to the point of seeing that Henry was not going to do it the cognitive route. Why?

Hilary, you will see in Chapter 13, was able to create small islands within her of (cognitive–emotional) knowledge, from which she could channel her defence against her attacking mother. Henry just did not process like that. It might be about permanent structure – personality or learning styles – or it might be a temporary deadening, but Henry could not form these island resources. So he was stuck. I was frustrated. He hated himself for being stuck. I wanted to rescue him and I could feel the potential of my irritation to further lower his self-esteem. The short time span of the ending was a (partly unconscious) attempt to force all of the issues. He and I were locked together. Only the shift in my supervisor unlocked us usefully.

I invited Henry to take control of the sessions. I could not force an ending, I told him. I could accompany him, but could not force the issue. Only Henry could be responsible. I let go. Within half an hour Henry's internal and largely unconscious processing responded. He could look at himself again. 'When I am in pain, my default position is (surly) teenager'. It is not that he needed to see that he was being a teenager. This does not matter a lot. It was that Henry could again stand to one side and access – and hence trust, albeit within limits – his processing, the *way* he does it, when in pain.

The result of making contact with the cut-off felt-sense of his pain and the concomitant regression (Gendlin, 1981, 1997) was that he could open up true sadness and the unthinkable anxiety of admitting that maybe he really was not happy with Jenny, however admirable she might be. To be truly unhappy is to be far more congruent. Whatever the outcome of Henry's relationship with Jenny and his child, he has reached a place where he can derive from the agonizing question properly existential meaning in life. Is it better to be loyal or fulfilled? Or is that not finally an actual dilemma for him?

## Process and Explanation

I want to end this study of Henry with an observation about the role of process awareness and the resulting interactions in constructing explanations of what happens in therapy. *Thinking about process* is to use a model of therapy, and hence a route to understanding. There are at least three possible explanations of what happened between me and Henry. The first I offer above.

The second might be that of some person-centred therapists with attachment to purist theory. It might simply be said that I had failed to accord Henry the core conditions by being judgemental, or by carelessly hijacking the flow of therapy. Well, this is not wholly wrong, of course. However, it is thin theory. Unlike the process account, it does not show that my process, Henry's process and my supervisor's process had an organic link which itself is to be trusted. At times we do just get it wrong, occasionally badly so. But more often our errors are rich with meaning. Process work, within ourselves and beyond, can contact this meaning. Process work is firstly a *thinking hard* about process, and then being willing to act in accordance with what is thought and recognized.

The third account comes typically from psychodynamic theory. It is transference and counter-transference. Was it not the case that I was acting out the role of Henry's father, lost, infuriating, rejecting? Was not my new-found permission a resolution of Henry's feelings about his father? Again, maybe there is some truth in this. From time to time I find thinking about transference really useful. Not on this occasion, though. To bolt for transference is in a way too safe. I miss the force of my irritation as real when I attribute it to counter-transference.

The model of therapy that thinks process is useful in that it opens up the parallels between theory and mental content, between therapist, supervisor and client, and finally between some elements of neuroscience and the everyday content of therapy. In the following chapter, we will revisit in some historical context the task of understanding person-centred process work.

## Further Reading

*The best ways into person-centred therapy and questions of process are contained in the Further Reading for the next chapter. The following two books offer important insights into how we learn through experience:*

Kolb, D. (1984) *Experiential Learning*. Englewood Cliffs, NJ, Prentice Hall.
Schön, D.A. (1987) *Educating the Reflective Practitioner*. San Francisco, Jossey-Bass.

# Part I
## Addressing Process Work

# 2

# What is Process in Person-Centred Therapy?

The classical, client-centred therapist will follow the client with care, seeking to understand and be led by the client, in the spirit of non-directivity (Merry, 1999, 2004). The experiential therapist will see herself as needing to follow the client's content for much of the time, but will change role at times to use her expertise, her fullness of grasp, of the client's process (Rennie, 1998, pp. 71–89). I believe that the client's process can be usefully addressed in person-centred therapy without taking the expert and directive stance of the experiential therapist.

This chapter will elaborate upon the basic idea of process. Some people have the ability to know and recognize process straight away; for others it is not easy. First, the case study of Maria will exemplify process as addressed within therapy. I link this to your own experience of everyday conversation. I then offer selected, brief sketches of the key points in the thought of a number of theorists from within the person-centred and experiential schools of therapy, in order to set my own thought in context. The final part of this chapter is a first statement of my own position. But first comes Maria.

The session with Maria shows not only what client and therapist process is, but demonstrates that the therapist has no choice but to face the choice about whether she intervenes at the level of process.

**Case 2.1  Maria**

Maria had been in therapy with me for about ten months. We developed a warm and trusting relationship over that time, and Maria felt free to begin to contact her vulnerabilities, as well as those emotions which had been forbidden by her father and her husband. She wanted to face some major life decisions, but was struggling to dare to say how she felt about her quality of life to those who mattered to her. She felt unheard. She saw that those around her might not want to hear her, but she also understood that she tended to expect others not to hear her. She had a knack of becoming a little invisible. This annoyed her. Yet we noted that she did not feel that she was invisible to me.

In the previous session, I had lost concentration on the time and had overrun by 15 minutes. (I have no clear view of the meaning of this.) At the beginning of the session, Maria said that she wanted to talk about what had happened when she got back out to her car. She had not had her watch with her that day. Only on seeing the car's clock did she realize that we had run over time. She was mortified. It must be her fault!

For a few minutes, we worked on her perception that she had taken full responsibility for what we both knew was my primary responsibility, to keep the boundaries of the session. I apologized for my error. She said that she felt within herself how difficult it was for her to let go of feeling responsible for others, and even of wanting to rescue them.

During the next 30 minutes or so, she moved across a number of subjects. I followed her, but would from time to time offer her my own perception of her. Near the end, she said that she felt that she had 'deliberately' moved from subject to subject and that this felt chaotic to her.

I was uncertain as to what was happening for her. Perhaps my failing to keep a time boundary had induced this. I spent a little time paying attention to my own feelings. I know that the 'its all my fault for being a bad counsellor' script would have been beguilingly self-punishing for me. I wondered if she felt angry with me. She said not. (But then it would have been something of an achievement for Maria to say she felt angry with me.) I became aware at this point that, in my listening over the period of 30 minutes, I had given her feedback as to how I saw her on a number of occasions.

On the surface, I could see that I was offering her my perceptions and experiences of her over against her own. Why did it feel to me strangely appropriate, but to Maria rather chaotic? Between us we had to wrestle our way towards a version of events that rang bells within her.

## Reflection

The piece of work with Maria had fallen into three parts. We had looked at how she had experienced her guilty surprise at having overrun time.

We then experienced a period of therapy, the content of which I can no longer remember. At the end of this, Maria had commented upon the fact that to her it had felt chaotic and between us, two puzzled people, we tried to make sense of what had been happening. The touchstone for this last movement was always what felt to make sense of the experience for Maria.

In the first movement, Maria had decided to work with a piece of her own processing: how, within her, she experienced the time problem and her relationship to it. What she brought to this work was the awareness that she was playing out a familiar scenario, and that she had played it out unconsciously until she had space and time to reflect upon it.

As she heard me reflect to her both the content and associated emotions of her experience, she went through a parallel experiencing, another version of the first. In the first experience, she was overwhelmed with guilt, and then with the sense that this was shockingly incongruent, out of kilter with her growing self-concept as a person who need not take responsibility for others. In talking about this experience, she paralleled it in her curiosity and annoyance that she had not escaped some old and familiar patterns. I had nothing to do but to remain with her own travelling self-awareness, watching it unfold before me.

In the second movement, the content is now lost to me. What stood out was that Maria experienced chaos, and I experienced a need to be as congruent with her as possible about how I saw her. Neither of us knew what was going on. The process was foremost, but neither client nor therapist was in expert role!

The third movement was a shared puzzlement. Maria began by noticing her sense of wandering aimlessly through themes. I then had a stark choice. Should I simply reflect what she was expressing, or should my focus be on my own experiencing? I chose the second. I cannot say that I can express why, or even claim that I was fully conscious of the decision. Yet it turned out to be creative. Neither of us knew why we were processing in a particular way, but we both opted to focus upon this.

The alternative would have been to opt to focus upon Maria's frame of reference rather than my own or a shared frame. There are times when it is logically impossible not to be directive at this level. It is likely, as here, that the therapist's choice will be made before she becomes fully aware of it. All that can be done is to share this choice with the client. I wanted Maria to be an equal partner with me at all times.

Our shared conclusion was that her chaos and my feedback constituted an experiment in congruence. An experiment in congruence was just where, in the previous session, Maria had reached. Could she congruently tell those whom she cared for that her present life would not do? Would they hear?

I have lost a grip on *how* we reached this version. If it came mainly from me, it was an interpretation and possibly bad person-centred therapy. If it came from the space between us, it was the fruit of two confused people thinking hard, and I guess that is OK.

# What is Process Work?

The client's process is the 'how' of her experiencing, the way she makes meaning out of life's raw data from the acts, sensations and functions of living. For Maria, her process was made up of:

- her initial reaction in her car to the fact that I had ended our session late;
- her emotion of guilt and her thinking about this reaction at the beginning of the next session;
- her moving from subject to subject in the second part of the session;
- her desire to notice this and then her sharing with me in reflecting upon it with puzzlement.

My own process was made up of:

- a hearing of her reaction in her car and a reflection of this so that she could make links to 'past patterns'. The links were either hers or were already in our shared frame of reference that makes up the history of our work together;
- A tracking of her work in the second part of the hour, with a sense that this was 'business as usual';
- A recognition that I was not actually behaving in a usual fashion, but was skewed towards feedback;
- A largely pre-conscious decision to address myself to this with Maria;
- A fully conscious decision to take responsibility for this and check out with her that what I was doing was OK.

---

**Personal Focus 2.1   Noticing process**

Recall a recent conversation that you have a keen memory of, can picture, or deliberately notice the process within the next extended conversation you have. It is more effective if the conversation has some emotional content;

Listen carefully to its content – the 'what'? of it;

Now move your attention from the 'what'? to the 'how'? of it;

Describe what you are noticing as the 'how'?, sometimes called the texture of the conversation. Check this against my description of my process with Maria above;

Notice that you have now transferred your attention from the 'what'? to the 'how'? of the words. What differences does this make to you?

Notice how the 'what'? and the 'how'? interweave, and inform each other;

> ▪ Allow yourself to imagine what difference it would make to draw the other person's attention to the process;
> ▪ What might be the benefits and the problems of this?

The whole subject of this book centres upon the question: is it person-centred to address the client's (and therapist's) process as well as the overt content and emotion of her work? I will argue in the coming chapters that process needs to be understood in terms of its relationship to the client's frame of reference, and thence to its embeddedness in phenomenological and existential perspectives.

My describing of Maria's process together with the simple question about how process can be addressed belies the maelstrom of passion that this debate has generated in the person-centred movement. To understand this, I will look briefly at the issues raised by David Rennie, Barbara Temaner Brodley and Laura Rice.

## Two Aspects of Process – The Work of David Rennie

Until 1998, the process-experiential approach to person-centred therapy was available in the learned books and articles of the likes of Alvin Mahrer, Les Greenberg and Laura Rice. The major exception was, of course, the popularized idea of focusing developed by Eugene Gendlin (1981) – see p. 22. In 1998, David Rennie published his own experiential approach as a midway position between Rogers and Gendlin. Its accessibility will guarantee that it will become a standard view.

For Rennie, process can be either reflexive or spontaneous. This is one of his major contributions. He sees humanity as characterized by its reflexivity. That is to say, we can think about thinking and feeling; we can feel about thinking and feeling. We are aware that we are aware and can work with this fact. For Rogers (1957c), spontaneity, free flow of process, is the key to healthy functioning. Rennie (2006) observes that clients also access what he terms *radical reflexivity*. That is, the client becomes aware of being self-aware. In so doing, she develops a conscious idea of her own agency and power. This too is an important step towards healing.

For Maria, there were times in her piece of work with me that she was spontaneously experiencing; at other times she was in reflexive mode. She felt guilty because she had run over time with me, a spontaneous experience. She had felt the sense of playing an old tape that she recognized. This is reflexive experience. However, spontaneity and reflexivity do not separate out so easily as this, for in reflecting she also generated for herself new and spontaneous experience: frustration, anger, embarrassment and thence a resolve to move on. The two modes can alternate swiftly in processing.

Therapists can then respond so as to point to process. This increases reflexive awareness in the client, but remains, if well done, empathic. Consider the two following responses to a client:

> I notice that as you talk about the sadness you feel at the way your boss treats you, you clench your fists.

> As you talk about the sadness you have at the way your boss treats you, you clench your fists. I wonder if you feel angry with him too.

The first of these is strictly phenomenologically accurate. It 'records' what happens physically, and what is being said at the time. The second is 'interpretative' just to the extent that it links the fist-clenching to a perhaps unacknowledged emotion. It is more deeply empathic. It is selective, but then anything that is said in therapy is selected out of the vast pool of all that might be said. (In all phenomenological work, there is a real tension between the aim to give all experience equal weight and the plain fact that this is a counsel of perfection.) It is a valid challenge to the client which would perhaps facilitate her awareness of unacknowledged or forbidden feelings such as anger. The two examples of process work above are embodiments of the core conditions yet the more 'interpretative' is also more deeply empathic.

Rennie's worked examples are informative. However, he speaks of process work in a way which I find unhelpful:

> This is the act of process *directing* that most clearly separates this expe-
> riential person-centred approach from the literal approach. When process
> directing, counsellors take charge. They assume the role of expert –
> an expert in process. In keeping with the experiential therapies, in this
> approach to person-centred counselling it is held that there are times when
> clients need help in dealing with themselves.
>
> (Rennie, 1998, p. 81)

If process work is seen as a type of empathy, then there is no need to think of a change of role for the counsellor from someone who is tracking the client's process in terms of the core conditions of relating, thence becoming an expert who steps in because the client needs help. There is real suspicion of process work by some practitioners – see for instance Jerold Bozarth (1998, p. 24) – and so those of us who advocate paying closer attention to the client's process need to stress that this does not necessarily involve a change of therapist role. The aim should be to maintain a constancy of role whether we are working with the client at the level of content or of process.

Rennie, then, raises a key point. Clients operate both spontaneously and reflexively; these two ends of a continuum operate in a multi-layered way. Reflexive process at one point also generates spontaneous process at another level. When Maria thinks about how she felt in the car, she can recall as memory her feelings then, but the act of recalling generates experience in the present thinking and feeling. It is this phenomenon of reflexive process leading to a parallel spontaneous process which, according to Rice (1974, 1984) and Greenberg *et al.* (1993), brings about change. In therapy, being in touch with content, feeling or process generates new, spontaneous emotion and cognition, which brings about change in the self-structure.

Rennie's contribution to the debate is to have developed some new thinking about the nature of spontaneity and reflexivity, suggesting that reflexivity is more important than Rogers noticed. However, he prejudices the debate about process work by attaching to it the notion that it requires the therapist to adopt a directive-expert role.

Brodley and Rice point to other key motifs on either side of the debate.

## Barbara Temaner Brodley and Laura North Rice

In 1990, Barbara Brodley published a paper in which she set out her perception of the differences between person-centred and experiential therapy. She raises a number of crucial issues. Before looking at them, a health warning! Brodley addresses almost exclusively the work of Eugene Gendlin. It is far from obvious why Gendlin should be seen as representative of process-orientation. He is perhaps the most overtly instrumentalist and directive of practitioners. Nevertheless, her characterization of person-centred therapy is important. She raises the following issues amongst others:

- Rogers' process conception of psychotherapy is a phenomenological analysis of client change, and not a set of instructions for therapist intervention;
- Rogers' process conception is therefore misunderstood if it changes the goals, attitude or behaviour of the therapist;
- Person-centred therapy addresses the whole person and not just their process;
- Experiential therapists see themselves as an expert on the client's process if not her content, and this is an inappropriate use of therapist power, violating a central tenet of Rogers' work.

In so saying, Brodley offers a useful challenge to Rennie's position, but misses the fact that there are process-orientated positions which do not have the characteristics of Rennie's.

In 1974, Laura Rice wrote an influential article about what she termed 'evocative empathy'. She puts the case that:

- Evocative empathy is the reflection of feeling in which the therapist's intention is to facilitate the client in 'a reprocessing of experience'. It is therefore not a vastly different technique, in the way that Gendlin's focusing is.

However, Rice does describe it as a technique. Rogers (1986b) is scathing of 'reflection as technique'. The re-processing of experience seems close to what I have described above as the client's movement between reflexive and spontaneous experience. The key issue here is that evocative empathy is a characteristic of therapist intention. Is this necessarily the case? Rice talks of 'targets of therapy', a phrase with which I am most uncomfortable. Where in this is the client's power?

- 'The basic assumption is that for any person there are some classes of experience that have never been adequately processed, and for some people, there are many such classes' (Rice, 1974, p. 293). This can of course be a general truth. It offers the therapist the chance to address each class of experience symptomatically, selectively and directively. This is certainly the direction of Rice's later work – see the latter part of Greenberg *et al.* (1993). However, it does not imply that the therapist should necessarily respond in this way. Work with symptoms is *prima facie* eclectic rather than person-centred.

- 'When evocative reflection is successful, it is as if the client goes back into the situation with a more or less deliberate suspension of his usual automatic construction' (Rice, 1974, p. 299). While I think that the client goes into new experience rather than returning to the old experience, what Rice is describing here is the client's own ability to work through her introjects. This can be the work of the actualizing tendency and not a directive therapist.

There is of course far more in the articles of both Brodley and Rice than I have selected here. These points serve to emphasize key issues.

## Focusing

Eugene Gendlin worked with Carl Rogers at the University of Chicago Counselling Centre from the 1950s onwards, until the latter left for California. His work was valued greatly by Rogers, but brought a very different slant to person-centred therapy. Gendlin was not only a psychologist but also a philosopher. As such he made two connected but separate contributions to theory. In his doctoral thesis (Gendlin, 1997) he explored the origins of meaning as bodily. (This will receive some attention in Chapter 10.) However, it is the practical spin-off from this which is of concern here. He developed a set of techniques which he called *focusing* (Gendlin, 1981; Purton, 2007).

Campbell Purton (2007, p. 8) characterizes focusing as a return to the client's experience. This is a close parallel to my own conviction that the client's process can get ignored in therapy. Gendlin begins by noting that experience is not (yet!) either a set of ideas or a set of emotions. It normally begins as, to use his key term, a *felt-sense*.

An example will illustrate the meaning of felt-sense. I recall going to my newsagents to ask for a copy of my Saturday newspaper, which they had apparently forgotten to deliver. I was told that, far from being an omission, this was deliberate, because I had not paid a bill for £10.32, which I had received four days previously! In short, I asked a few questions to clarify my understanding of the situation, and then left, saying what I would not require them to be my newsagents in future. I crossed the road and noted a sense of pleasure that I had responded effectively and congruently. 'That's how to do it, Richard!'

However, that is the short version. What really happened took place in my guts. I realized as I talked to the manageress that the absent newspaper was not an accident, but punitive! Inside me, a warmth emerged. At first I took no notice, but over a period of three or four seconds felt the beginnings of anger. I consulted it. It was there. I was angry. A little reflection told me why. I moved coldly and with calculation to confront her. As I spoke, the cool glow of anger hovered in my lower gut. I knew that if I allowed the line of it, its top, to rise up in me, quite literally, then I might lose control verbally. As I crossed the road afterwards, I felt triumphant. Then, for the few minutes in which I walked home, the red glow of it swamped me. I wanted to tear her limb from limb, to dissect and obliterate her. I arrived at home, and gradually let go of the lurking fury. It had astonished me. So real! Yet, not part of what I meant to do.

Focusing is mental technique which helps people locate first the gut-awareness, the felt-sense. Then the sense can gradually be named and becomes an emotion. Emotions do not happen fully formed (Greenberg *et al.*, 1993) but emerge gradually from a dialogue between the underlying schemes (see Chapter 13) and current experience.

The challenge of Gendlin is this. Is it compatible with the person-centred approach to conduct these pieces of directive therapy within the broader context of the client's free-flow. Each therapist must decide for herself. However, even if it is not, what can the therapist learn from Gendlin's focusing *theory*, which can influence her engagement with the client productively?

## The Person-Centred Rigidity

While the issues raised by the above thinkers may look matters for interesting debate, the degree of bitterness generated by this has at times been notorious (Thorne, 1992, pp. 90–9). To any who read the work of Carl Rogers closely, it must be evident that he was committed to facilitating personal freedom and personal power. This is for me poignantly the case in Rogers' writings on marriage and its alternatives:

> When a partnership is based on growing, evolving choice, when its interpersonal politics is free from the desire to control, it develops in a unique,

idiosyncratic way. It shows that when two people are openly and freely endeavoring to be themselves, highly individual patterns emerge. It is not a model, it cannot be copied, but provides much food for thought.

(Rogers, 1978, pp. 205–6)

Although he writes here of marriage, he could have written the same words about the therapeutic relationship.

Rogers invites us to taste, to investigate, to experience. He was an outstanding and committed empirical researcher. Indeed, he asks us to adopt his view of the counsellor's role – at the very heart of his thinking – not as theory but as hypothesis (Rogers, 1951, pp. 35–6). 'Try it for yourself and see how it is!'

I therefore record my strong reservation concerning what I take to be a conservative and rigid element in the thinking of some person-centred practitioners. This book is an invitation to the freedom of moving away from being what might ironically be called 'dogmatic person-centredness'.

The person-centred and experiential family of therapies has at times been marked by much vitriol about the issues briefly illustrated above. In 2000, Pete Sanders tried to bring about an outbreak of peace, by a careful description of what is core to all members of the family, and what is secondary and so differences we can agree to disagree about. I have found his Chicago position statement invaluable in setting out my own position, in practice as well as in the act of theorizing.

## The Chicago 2000 Position Statement

In an attempt to negotiate a major outbreak of peace within the person-centred and experiential movement, Pete Sanders offered a hugely important paper to the Fifth International Conference on Person-Centred and Experiential Psychotherapy in Chicago in June 2000. (See also Lietaer, 2002.) His position statement, which he encourages person-centred practitioners and organizations to adopt, describes two sets of criteria by which to judge whether a practitioner is person-centred. The primary set are non-negotiable:

---

### Box 2.1   Primary principles of person-centred therapies

- The primacy of the actualizing tendency – it is a therapeutic mistake to believe, or act upon the belief, that the therapeutic change process is *not* motivated by a client's actualizing tendency.
- Assertion of the necessity of therapeutic conditions (1957a, 1959) and therapeutic behaviour based on *active inclusion* of these – it is a therapeutic mistake to *exclude* any of the conditions. *Passive* inclusion, assuming that such conditions are always

present in all relationships is also insufficient. This primary principle, which declares the paramount importance of the relationship in person-centred therapy, requires active attention to the provision of these conditions.

Primacy of the non-directive attitude *at least* at the level of content but not necessarily at the level of process. It is permissible for the therapist to be an 'expert' *process*-director – it is a therapeutic mistake to direct the content of a client's experience either explicitly or implicitly.

It is clear from Box 2.1 that process-orientated therapy as I describe it here is conducive with the primary conditions. Indeed, the permission to use process direction in an expert role is, as I have said above, unnecessary. However, I note that the inability of any therapist to avoid selection and hence at some level directivity blurs the edges between the classical and the experiential approaches rather more than either Sanders or Rennie countenance.

However, when we turn to the secondary principles, those which we might expect to be more akin to classical client-centred therapy, the current approach is less prone to 'pick and choose' than might be expected. Rather it challenges some of the presuppositions inherent in some readings of the secondary principles.

---

**Box 2.2   Secondary principles of person-centred therapies**

Autonomy and the client's right to self determination – it is a therapeutic mistake to violate the internal locus of control.

Equality, or non-expertness of therapist – it is a therapeutic mistake to imply that the therapist is an expert in the direction of the content and substance of the client's life.

The primacy of the non-directive attitude and intention in its absolute and pure form as elaborated by, for example Barbara Brodley. Shlien (2000) suggests that such a principle be called *inherently non-directive* – it is a therapeutic mistake to wrest control of change process from client's actualizing tendency in any way whatsoever.

Sufficiency of the therapeutic conditions proposed by Rogers (1957a, 1959) – it is a therapeutic mistake to *include* other conditions, methods or techniques.

Holism – it is a therapeutic mistake to respond to only a part of the organism.

Process work is indeed selective of that to which the therapist pays attention. It is a category error to think that classical work is not. In classical work there is preference to choose content over process, as a matter of habit or principle; yet this is still a choice, and is directive, for the classical therapist deflects the client from the process-oriented aspects of her own frame of reference. I will suggest that within the limits of this logical conundrum process work can occur as a result of the therapeutic dyad being directed towards process by the client's actualizing tendency. That is to say, when process work is part of the language of working, the client can often sense when she needs to pay attention to the 'how' rather than the 'what' of her being. In consequence, the therapist is no more in an expert role than in classical work.

In the same way, process work need not wrest control from the client. There is always a to and fro between therapist and client. All therapist interventions from within their own frame of reference are part of this to-ing and fro-ing. In Rogers' own work, this sort of intervention varied between 4 per cent and 22 per cent of interventions. It is to underestimate grossly the power of the client to see all interventions from the therapist's frame of reference as wresting control from the client (Villas-Boas Bowen, 1996). Thus process work need not violate the sufficiency of the therapeutic conditions.

The last of the secondary principles – holism – is a clear plea for process work. To decline to address the client's process is to fail to respond to the whole of the organism.

The Chicago 2000 position statement serves to demonstrate that process work need not be as heterodox as is often supposed.

## An Initial Position

In the light of the controversy and polarization within the person-centred movement, I want to set out the following key points as the basis of my own practice, suggesting that it can be both process-orientated and still true to the necessity and sufficiency of the six conditions of therapy:

- As the client's process is an aspect of her frame of reference, way of being, then addressing it much resembles empathy. Indeed, it can be deeply empathic, but empathy with aspects of the client that are not fully expressed or yet in focus. This suggests that process work can be seen as relational in character. Far from being a technique, it is part of the repertoire of relating which is represented by the necessary and sufficient conditions of therapy (Rogers, 1957a).
- As the client is always 'in process', then it is always the case that the therapist is faced with a choice as to whether to respond to, to focus upon, the client's process or the client's content. Process and content exist simultaneously, and so giving equal weight to all aspects of the client is often difficult,

sometimes impossible. At this basic level, all person-centred therapists are directive because they have no choice but to choose.

- Clients move from the reflexive to the spontaneous end of their own repertoire of responses. It is possible of course to be highly directive of this. However, it is also possible to trust the client to know her own need of where to focus attention. This was the case with Maria.
- Rogers' process conception does not require that the therapist respond by changing her fundamental attitude. Process work can be 'tool-like' or it can be an expression of the fundamental person-centred attitude. It is an activity that can express a way of being and instantiate the core conditions of therapy.
- The quality of process work is not fixed by the verbal interactions with process *per se* but by the fundamental attitudinal stance of the therapist.
- The client's process is one aspect of her frame of reference. If I discount process, I discount part of my client. I can engage process when I grapple with the phenomenological nature of therapy.
- To the extent that person-centred therapy is an existential therapy, the basic principles of existentialism, such as the fact and nature of authentic living, for example, will stand over against the client's frame of reference. Frankel and Sommerbeck (2007) have indeed pointed out that from 1957 there was a real shift in Rogers' own practice, in that he was more willing in the name of congruence to speak from his won frame of reference, over against that of the client.
- Process is one aspect of the whole person. To minimize it is to move away from a holistic approach to the client.
- It is not the case, as *per* Rennie, that the client is the expert on her content, and the therapist upon her process (Rennie, 1998, p. 2). Rather the client is the expert upon *her* content and *her* process, for they are aspects of her frame of reference and meaning, and so are incontestable in principle. However, therapists may feel that they have some expertise in the nature of content and process in general. Consequently, there is no need for the process-orientated therapist to be any more in expert role than the classical client-centred therapist.
- As with my interaction with Maria, the therapist sometimes responds to client process from her spontaneous self. This is an aspect of a larger relationship and not of an isolated therapeutic moment.
- Evocative empathy can be either a tool, a technique, or it can be a seeking to know and understand the client while trusting in actualizing tendency to use the evocative response for her own good.
- A client's process is fundamentally trustworthy. In engaging with it, a therapist can let it guide her.
- When there are two people in the room, there are three frames of reference. The shared one comes in part from that which is jointly known, embedded in the history of the work, and partly from the out-of-awareness interaction of two people-in-process.

## Moving to Process Work

Pete Sanders notes in his Foreword to the first edition of this book that this is for some 'a contentious and challenging book'. There are two reasons for this. The first is that the central tenets of the book have to be both argued out and then communicated experientially.

The second concerns the reader's feelings about the implications of these arguments for her own practice. For some, process-orientation may be refreshing, and even a relief. For others, it will be of genuine interest and can be read sympathetically, perhaps because it is wholly alien to their own classically based practice and, as wholly alien, is strangely safe. For yet others there may be a sense of disorientation. That which is known and familiar and strongly held and secure is open to challenge, not by an Alvin Mahrer or even a David Rennie, but by an author who is arguing that the integration of theory and awareness of philosophical implications is to be combined with a new practical stance of working actively with process while attempting to remain faithful to the six conditions of therapy.

I invite the reader to be in touch with her own feelings through the use of an image:

---

**Personal Focus 2.2   Imaging change**

▪ Imagine that you are travelling on a difficult journey. It may be across a snow field on skis, or through a forest, or even sailing along the coast line;

▪ As you journey, note what markers you use to discover where you are. What are these markers, signs, aids to navigation?

▪ How do you use them? What are your feelings about the journey?

▪ One day, you notice that the all-too-familiar markers have subtly changed. How?

▪ What feelings does this promote in you? What range of feelings?

▪ Use this image as you choose, perhaps a number of times.

▪ What does it say to you about meeting new markers, patterns, challenges in your practice of therapy?

---

In the next chapter, we move on to a closer appreciation of the client in process.

## Further Reading

Baker, N. (2007) *The Experiential Counselling Primer*. Ross-on-Wye, PCCS Books.

Nick Baker's thoughtful approach to being experiential does justice to the Canadian, American and European experiential therapists, while retaining a flavour all of its own.

This book represents an attempt to keep a balance between the directive and non-directive, and so is in the same spirit as the present volume.

Merry, T. (1999) *Learning and Being in Person-Centred Counselling.* Ross-on-Wye, PCCS Books.

Perhaps the most lively and engaged overview of person-centred counselling, in particular for those who are in training or newly qualified. It has plenty of exercises with which the reader can help along the internal processes of growth.

Rennie, D. (1998) *Person-Centred Counselling: An experiential approach.* London, Sage.

The crispest of those books that is definitely experiential. A valuable resource, particularly in thinking through why some therapists want to be directive of process. It should, however, be complemented by Baker (2007), who is experiential but less directive.

Sanders, P. (ed.) (2004) *The Tribes of the Person-Centred Nation: An introduction to the schools of therapy related to the person-centred approach.* Ross-on-Wye, PCCS Books.

This book provides a superbly well-constructed overview of the many variants within the person-centred movement, in the voices of a number of mature practitioners. Its layout and way of presenting material is novel and very useful indeed.

Sanders, P. (2006) *The Person-Centred Counselling Primer.* Ross-on-Wye, PCCS Books.

The best introduction to the classical, client-centred approach. Rich and extremely well-written, it describes itself as 'concise, accessible and comprehensive', and it is. It is one of a series of seven *Primers* from PCCS Books. All are valuable resources.

# 3

# The Client in Process

In his (1957c) paper entitled 'A Process Conception of Psychotherapy', Carl Rogers asked the question: by what process does the personality change? As he began to seek a method for his research, he was struck by the lack of research into process at that time in many disciplines. It was as if science were more interested in taking a slice through a phenomenon at one point in time only. Rogers did not want to know just how the client was at any one point in time, but rather how that change across time might be observed and described. His seven stages of psychotherapy, together with its expansion in his (1959) paper, is described by him as phenomenological observation combined with low-level abstractions so that from these can be formulated testable hypotheses. There has followed from this work much research into the outcome of client-centred therapy and of the necessary and sufficient conditions of therapy.

Rogers' aim in his 1957 paper was clearly to promote psychotherapy outcome research. He certainly gives no warrant to experiential therapists to engage in process work.

The purpose of this chapter is therefore not to claim that Rogers particularly sanctions process work. Rather, it is to examine the claim that, as soon as therapy is seen as a process at all, then the question of how the therapist addresses that process is inescapable.

## Two Practice Observations

Near the end of his life, Carl Rogers wrote,

> What I wish is to be at her side, occasionally falling a step behind, occasionally a step ahead when I can see more clearly the path we are on, and taking a leap ahead only when guided by my intuition.
> (Rogers, 1986a, cited in Kirschenbaum and Henderson, 1990a, p. 150)

Some 12 years later, the Belgian therapist and academic, Germain Lietaer, noted,

It is possible for a therapist to be process-directive in a truly dialogic and democratic way. Offering the 'Rogerian' attitudes and focusing on the experiential world of the client – to me the core aspects of the experiential paradigm – merge into a highly influential process…yet at its best it is always a process in which the organismic awareness of the person functions as the ultimate guide.

(Lietaer, 1998 in Thorne and Lambers, 1998, pp. 70–1)

I suggest that Rogers' valuing of his own intuition is of major importance to process work. It is part of Rogers' congruence in his being with the client that there are times when he sees further ahead than the client. The image that occurs to me is of two people in a dark tunnel, each equipped with a flashlight. From time to time, the therapist is able to shine the beam further ahead than the client. (On many more occasions it is the client who can do this. In any case, what is actually seen in the pool of light is always for the client to determine.)

When the therapist's intuition leads, it begs two questions: why and how?

If Rogers' intuition is as trustworthy as the above quotation suggests, then he is in deep contact with the client, understanding her always tentatively but occasionally with insight which goes beyond her own focused awareness. There are many reasons why Rogers might develop a productive hunch, one worth the risk. He is not inhibited in the journey forwarded by the same defence-patterns as the client. He brings his own experience of other work, and can see the client's world not only from the client's own frame of reference but also from that of an experienced therapist. He has available to him some elements of the relationship that are not within the client's awareness. He is aware of transferential content, an awareness which is often denied by the client. Rogers is similarly aware of the client's process. In his famous interview with Kathy (Rogers, 1977), Kathy gets to the point of having told Rogers of her presenting problem, and then she stops. There is a silence. Kathy feels that she is unwilling to say more. Rogers not only touches this feeling in her but extends this to encompass all of her relationships – just so far and no further. This is a leap of intuition on his part, but a leap that is based on his knowledge over many years about how clients process their feelings and the expression of them. Rogers can trust his intuition because he has a storehouse of practical wisdom about possible client behaviour and underlying process. He has expertise about parallel process and countertransference, but not about Kathy's meaning or process. These he checks out with her.

If that is *why* he can trust his intuition, then *how* does he do this? The basic answer must be with an awareness that the leap forward is also tentative. He must avoid using any privileged knowledge as a source of power over his client. He may step out ahead, but then must await the client's judgement upon what he has done.

Yet, not only is it possible for process work to be faithful to the client's autonomy and frame of reference, but the very act of working with the client's process can be an engagement with her organismic valuing process. In the act of engaging, the therapist is guided by the client and her process. This I illustrate with the case study of John, a young man suffering from panic attacks.

---

**Case 3.1 John**

John had been afraid of his puritanical but well-meaning father. His father's disapproval had been a childhood theme for him and his two brothers. He knew that he was loved but felt, deep down, that if he failed at anything then that was to betray himself and his father. His father was an accomplished engineer. John, an accounts manager with a local furniture store, did not live up to his father's skilfulness. For years he avoided manual work. Now in his forties, he recognized that this was an unfulfilled element of himself, and tried to get into home woodwork. Visits to the local store to buy materials could bring on a panic attack. The very fact of things going wrong in the home would reduce him to rage.

He felt his feelings viscerally, but they were misattributed. He was still subject to his father's fierce gaze during a panic attack; when confronted with a task to be done, he was still living out his own rage at the unfairness of his parental home.

Unlike some clients, he was not cut off from his feeling processes, but his strong conditions of worth caused him to symbolize his life-meanings inappropriately.

After a number of weeks of therapy, John presented the panic attacks as his main felt-problem. In careful listening, I noticed his muscular tension, his holding of himself from within, as it were. I reflected this back as both tense and fearful and so, so tiring. John first began to experience his panic more fully, more physically – that is, as sensation rather than 'the desire to freeze or run'. Careful and time-consuming dwelling with this helped John to make links to his experiences with his father in childhood and early teens. 'I never could do anything right for him.' 'Yes, he loved me, and I suppose I love him, but for Dad love is never enough.' 'I felt paralysed by his demands for perfection.'

The linking of his bodily awareness of panic to his awareness of his father only gradually became a conscious element of John's self-knowing, but throughout our work I tracked it in him. Gradually, I noted that the pent-up rage began to be symbolized more accurately as sadness (itself still a defence against rage) for his father. It was to be a while before the 'sad' feelings in the pit of the stomach became even more accurately felt and symbolized as anger, for to be angry with Dad was never safe.

*Yet my client had a wisdom of his own within his body. He had a capacity to engage viscera and meaning. He had the resource to 'find' it true experience.* The panic attacks subsided. The fence even got mended. But above all John moved on to deal consciously with his relationship, past and present, with his father.

## Reflection

As John's therapist, I saw one of my chief tasks as being aware of the whole of him, including his body, his musculature, his breathing, his stomach. I could *see* the physical manifestations of his incongruence. I needed to respond to his experience of suppressing experience. At first, the insight from this guided my own responding and tracking of all that John was – and I was never fully sure of what I was seeing, particularly in the early days of our work, for getting to know the client is about learning how they process as well as the more personal elements of knowing. Gradually, I felt that his experiencing of his body could be offered back to his conscious awareness. There is always a balancing act between spontaneity and reflexivity. Once or twice I reined back the desire to 'experiment' with John. He would emphasize his physical awareness naturally, I reminded myself. Often, my 'noticing' was enough. Very occasionally I would ask him to be aware and even to repeat an action – but this has to be done infrequently and with constant checking out of permission from the client. I acted here with healthy self-suspicion.

Process work is another aspect of the tension between spontaneity and reflexivity. If I avoid the client's process, so will she. I want her to be in spontaneous process. At times this will mean risking making the fact and content of that processing reflexively known. This is not a teaching tactic, or a crass sort of experiment. It is acknowledging that the client's frame of reference is the whole of her being at any moment, and thus empathy is also a shared struggle to know the elements of process which are out of awareness as well as those of which the client is aware.

I recall a passage about the reflection of feelings from one of Rogers' last writings:

From my point of view as a therapist, I am *not* trying to 'reflect feelings'. I am trying to determine whether my understanding of the client's inner world is correct – whether I am seeing it as he or she is experiencing it at this moment. Each response of mine contains the unspoken question, 'Is this the way it is for you?'

(Rogers, 1986b, in Kirschenbaum and Henderson, 1990a, p. 127)

Person-Centred process work is a struggle to understand actively, not to interfere. What is added is the fact that the experience and meanings of the client are often exhibited by her body, her inner experiences which may be out of her awareness. As I struggle to understand my client's process, she too may become more reflexively aware of it.

I note that some clients use this reflexive awareness extensively; it can become a major metaphor of their own story. Others return it swiftly to the edge of awareness, sometimes to be denied, but far more often to be briefly and spontaneously consulted. What my clients do with their awareness of their process I have to entrust to their own actualizing tendency.

The clients' felt-sense of their need to engage process is an integral aspect of their frame of reference.

---

**Personal Focus 3.1   Contacting your processing preferences**

- Imagine that you are feeling angry with someone close to you. You are talking about this with a friend.
- Many of us are faced with the dilemma of how to engage anger. Do you want to feel it more keenly and tell the other person that you are angry with them, or are you more likely to want to bury it down again and avoid further disturbance?
- As you talk about your anger with a friend, how do you experience that anger? Does it intensify or decrease?
- As you reach the end of a period of focusing on your anger, does it return to the edge of your awareness, even more repressed perhaps, or do you feel it more keenly?
- Does focusing on your anger in the presence of an empathetic friend tend to lead you to act on it or to let go of it?
- How does this relate to what you consciously want to do with your anger?

*I postulate that for each client there will be very different patterns, and complex ones at that, about the original anger, what is experienced of anger in recollection, any feelings of incongruence between this awareness and willingness to face the anger with the other person, and the preferred way of processing that anger. The therapist needs to trust the processing of the client. It may lead to a freer flow of emotion and keener awareness. It may be part of a long and rugged path to the dissolution of deeply held incongruences. But above all trust the process.*

# Process Work and the Client's Frame of Reference

[The therapist has the purpose] of providing deep understanding and acceptance of the attitudes consciously held at this moment by the client as he
explores step by step into the dangerous areas he has been denying to
consciousness.

(Rogers and Dymond, 1954, p. 13)

In this early text, Rogers is making the link between the phenomenological
approach in general and the fact that the client works through her repression
via an acceptance of the contents of the current frame of reference. That which
is repressed is not consciously available to the client. It is certainly not the job
of the therapist, *qua* expert, to declare what this unconscious content is, nor
is it necessary for the client always to grasp through her own journeying the
whole of this content. However, for some clients a making-conscious-by-the-
client-in-process (as distinct from making conscious through the interpretation
of the therapist) can be a major element in the journey. Rogers believes that
the areas which are denied become available through the current awareness of
the client, as long as the six conditions of therapy are in place.

The question then can focus upon the meaning for us of the term 'frame of
reference'. This has a number of meanings. It can indicate a general view of
life, a *Weltanschauung*, a way of constructing the personal world. This endures
over time, changing only slowly. It corresponds very broadly to the notion of
the self-concept. However, 'frame of reference' also connotes the moment-
by-moment awareness of the client. In early days in counselling practice, one
of the commonest faults is to reflect back too much of what has been said a
couple of minutes previously, and is now past. When this happens, the client
is ripped untimely from her current frame of reference into a past frame, gone
some seconds or minutes before.

But what are the possible contents of this frame of reference? The content of
the client's conscious, reflexive awareness is obviously one aspect of her frame
of reference. Rogers both offers and requires a broader definition of awareness
than this. He was influenced by Gestalt psychology and by the work of Kurt
Lewin. Both argue that human beings must be seen as whole systems, in which
the interrelationships of the parts are crucial:

The real task [in psychology] is to investigate the structural properties of a
given whole, ascertain the relations of subsidiary wholes, and determine the
boundaries of the system with which one is dealing.

(K. Lewin, in Ellis, 1938. Cited imperfectly, Perls, 1973, p. 326)

Rogers clearly sees the human mind not as a unitary monad, a single system,
but as self-conscious, conscious and repressed areas, perhaps constituting a

number of subsystems, and certainly involving an interplay of thinking, feeling and bodily awareness.

Thus, in his filmed work with Kathy, Rogers (1977) is aware at a deeply empathic level that he has access to that which she is holding out of her own conscious awareness. He notes the moistening of the rims of her eyes. In making this link – 'I can see this in your eyes' – he facilitates a radical change of level and structure of awareness in Kathy. This is process work.

The client's frame of reference includes that which is self-consciously known, that which is passively but openly known, some elements at least of repressed material, Gendlin's 'felt sense' and a whole range of body states, some of which correspond to mental states. The moment-by-moment frame of reference is a complex of subsystems, to which only the client – if anyone – can have unmediated access. Some parts of any frame of reference correspond to the reflexive pole – what I know I know and feel – while others correspond to the spontaneous pole – what I experience but do not conceptualize, not even as formed emotion. Empathy can engage at any point on this continuum. The greater the spontaneous-type content of the frame of reference, the more proper it is to call any therapist response process-orientated, because the therapist will be engaging empathically with the whole organism who is the client, and not just the reflexive, conscious elements.

## Process Work and the Six Conditions of Therapy

Once it is seen that the client's process is one aspect of her frame of reference, and that to engage with it is therefore legitimate, it can clearly be seen that process work does not *sui generis* violate the necessity and sufficiency of the core conditions of therapy (Rogers, 1957a). Because the six conditions of therapy refer to a *quality* of relationship, it is clear that there is a *prima facie* case for addressing process as well as content.

Rogers (1959) summarizes the structure of the theory of personality and therapeutic change which it sets out. Understanding this structure will help us to distinguish between process work which embodies the core conditions of therapy from process work which is essentially not person-centred. This structure is typical of Rogers, the scientist. It is a deductive chain – a short sequence based on the formula 'If X, then Y: if Y then Z'. Rogers sets out his deductive chain thus:

IF {the six conditions of therapy} THEN {a process begins}
IF {the therapeutic process} THEN {constructive therapeutic change}.

This chain implies the necessity and sufficiency of the six conditions. The chain only holds if the six conditions necessarily and sufficiently bring about constructive therapeutic change. Process work departs from this and enters the realm of experiential psychotherapy just when therapist interventions are constructed to *manufacture* the process so that only the second line of the chain adheres. Process intervention is legitimately person-centred when it embodies the six conditions.

This sounds simple enough as a schema. Unfortunately it is not. Rogers points to two aspects of process. Process is change, in that this change releases the client into a new way of being. However, the very process that engenders the change is also the goal of that change. The fully functioning person is not someone who has reached a fixed point, but someone who is able to be in constant flow. Rogers (1957c) puts it thus:

> In general, the process moves from a point of fixity, where all the elements and threads described above are separately discernible and separately understandable, to the flowing peak moments of therapy in which all these threads become inseparably woven together. In the new experiencing with immediacy which occurs at such moments, feeling and cognition interpenetrate, self is subjectively present in the experience, volition is simply the subjective following of a harmonious balance of organismic direction. Thus, as the process reaches this point the person becomes a unity of flow, of motion. He has changed, but what seems most significant, he has become an integrated process of changingness.
>
> (Rogers, 1957c, in Rogers, 1967, p. 158)

Rogers (1959) expresses the matter more succinctly: There is no clear distinction between process and outcome. Items of process are simply differentiated aspects of outcome (Rogers, 1959 in Kirschenbaum and Henderson, 1990a, p. 241). In short, the process which brings about change subsists also in the outcomes of that change. I change by experiencing change, until I am flexible enough to risk being in constant process, no longer fixedly defended.

This may at first sight seem paradoxical. It is not. Rogers hypothesizes that as a result of the incongruence between the self and experience which stems from the frustration of the child's need for positive regard, there sets in a defence system which remains stable only as long as the discrepancies between the self and experience are not symbolized accurately. This defence system has the quality of rigidity or fixity. This is the very opposite of the process which is the middle term in Rogers' chain. Therapy often involves an initial breakdown of this defensive system. Rogers distinguishes three stages of this: a growing set of discrepancies in behaviour; the experience of feeling threatened as the defences fail; a process of breakdown and disorganization which precedes re-integration (Rogers, 1959, in Kirschenbaum and Henderson, 1990a, pp. 247–9).

In other words, fluent processing, both spontaneous and reflexive, is a key quality of healthy living. In dysfunction this is partly, even wholly, lost. In therapy, it is restored to some degree. The quality of relationship allows the client to experience flow because the therapist is able to accord the core conditions. The process is also inherent in the six conditions, to the extent that the therapist, necessarily more congruent than the client, embodies this flow of experience.

It is perhaps unique to person-centred therapy that the aims of the therapeutic relationship, the process of therapy as experienced by the client, and the goals and outcomes of therapy are essentially the same – a way of being.

Rogers has described in a number of places what it is like to be fully functioning. This would be the ultimate goal for our clients. However, it is part of the logic of that goal that it cannot be given, but must be found, for it is about *self*-actualization. The therapist must trust in the actualizing tendency, because this trust by therapist and client alike is a necessary condition of the outcome. Therefore any process work which artificially seeks to create experience within the middle term of Rogers' chain violates this key person-centred principle.

However, any process work which embodies in a genuine relationship the core conditions and helps the client to experience more fully their own, native processing, does not violate this principle.

Later on, in Chapter 13, we will look at the work of Garry Prouty and Margaret Warner in their work with people with psychosis. I will argue that this work with deeply disturbed clients has much to teach us about more everyday work. Here is a case in point. Prouty and Warner have, in different ways, developed ways of thinking about client process which has the specific aim of putting the client back in touch with her process (Prouty) or of considering the client's process so as better to understand her meaning (Warner). Working with process is at the cutting edge of person-centred theory.

## Spontaneity, Reflexivity and the Actualizing Tendency

We return to reflect further upon John.

John's body had had a wisdom of its own. Although the symptoms were very unpleasant to John, he had managed to express his conflicted feelings as panic. He had learned at least to give some attention to that which was denied focused awareness. It is useful to see the presenting problem, even when it is rather 'physical', as a manifestation of the client's actualizing tendency. John's body was just 'good enough' in expressing as panic the underlying relational conflict.

In therapy, John had come to experience the conflicted relationship in a more focused and reflexive fashion, by paying attention to his own process at the time that, out of awareness, he judged to be appropriate.

John and I were in constant dialogue. I had a real sense that the physiological processes were spontaneous expressions of his anxiety. I could empathize by struggling to understand his body as much as his story and feelings. As with any aspect of the client's frame of reference, I made delicate judgements about when to reflect these processes. The dialogue was between a reflexive awareness in me and a process of organismic evaluation in John. His process constantly assessed when he could become aware of his process. This evaluation was, I believe, in terms of safety. John needed to begin to experience his own body in such a way that he could offer it, his embodied and out-of-awareness processes, enough acceptance to derive from it a meaning which could be carried forward. This organismic evaluation of subjective and largely unconscious safety is as much an aspect of the client's work with his own process as it is with his emotions.

As a therapist, it is my task both to accept the process myself and to reflect it in a way that is what Lietaer calls 'democratic'. That is, I strive to reflect firmly enough to be hearable, and softly enough so as to give the client a choice about hearing.

As human beings we move constantly along a continuum between spontaneity and reflexivity. At times we need to experience ourselves in a free flow of process. We also need to reflect upon our experiencing. Therapy also includes a moving from one point on this continuum to another.

## Key Themes

The two central claims of this chapter are:

1. It is part of healthy living and good therapy that the client can move from free experiencing to careful reflection upon that experience. Experience is both conscious and non-conscious, because we are fully embodied beings. Whatever happens in focused awareness is a small part of our experiencing. Person-Centred therapy is at its most holistic (Sanders, 2000, secondary principle five) when it engages with the totality of the client's experience.
2. In engaging with the process-component of the client's frame of reference the therapist, far from becoming more directive, needs to trust the client's actualizing tendency in guiding him in the way that he engages. This meeting with the client's process is more complex, and at a micro-skills level might from time to time be directive, just to the extent that the client's process is out of the client's focused awareness. Yet, the degree of directivity can be very low. It is directive to notice my client's breathing and to reflect that. Indeed, it can alter the way he breathes. It is also directive to refuse to notice, to reflect, to engage.

There is, I suspect, a complex relationship between spontaneity and reflexivity on the one hand, and the decision to engage a client's process on the other. It would be possible to catalogue a large number of patterns of interplay between these components of therapy. In limited space, three examples will suffice:

---

### Box 3.1 Not interrupting the client

When my client is fluently engaged with her feelings or with her narrative, then I would be interrupting her were I to engage myself with underlying processing.

---

The actualizing tendency is a native wisdom within the client by which she can, over a period of time, seek to reduce the incongruence between aspects of her self-concept and her organismic need to feel, experience, express and accept her emotions and linked cognitions. When a client seems to be engaged with her own feelings (or cognitions, sometimes) then it is likely that her process is in healthy function. I may wish to draw this to her attention. Clients need to see in full consciousness at times that they are functioning well, for this can challenge those unhealthy scripts that say, I never get in touch with myself. However, as a generality, I would consider it a high risk to turn fluently spontaneous functioning into reflexive functioning.

Engaging the client's process is always a risk. Be aware of therapy as including a risk assessment. This is not just a quality of the more directive therapists. Carl Rogers, in making the bridge between Kathy's withdrawing from him and from other men, is taking a risk. It is the risk of interrupting her stuckness. Similarly, to have refused to do this would also have been a risk. We must engage this paradox.

---

### Box 3.2 A choice of interventions

When one of the most marked figures of my perception of a client is that her overt communication and her body state are incongruent, then I have a choice as to whether I focus my attention upon the one or the other. I cannot escape this choice.

---

Rogers believed that the six conditions of therapy (Rogers, 1957a) were sufficient to bring about such change as would reduce the incongruence between the client's self-concept and her true needs. If this is true, then it is the case that when the therapist perceives the client as incongruent, there is a real choice as to whether this should be challenged. It is not necessary to challenge the incongruence by noticing it, and yet it might be expedient to do this.

In the moment with Kathy alluded to above, Rogers clearly chooses to engage Kathy's process, and this challenges her to face the gap that she is manifesting, the gap between her desire to be intimate and her fear of intimacy.

The therapist's choice is logically always present, but in practice it is the therapist's intuition which allows him to perceive the process that might be engaged.

I conjecture that an experienced therapist monitors client process constantly, but that this spontaneous activity is normally only at the edge of awareness. From time to time the therapist will experience the process as becoming interesting, obvious or even tantalizing. It moves from ground to figure. The therapist cannot have self-conscious control of when this switch of frame of reference happens. We trust ourselves, for here we have no alternative. Intuition is likely to be a fast, largely out-of-awareness process of monitoring and deducing.

---

**Box 3.3   Increased reflexivity**

Especially in the latter part of a long-term, therapeutic relationship, I notice that many clients seem to have learned to move from the spontaneous to the reflexive, and moreover have developed a clear view, I suspect as a felt-sense, of when they need to make this move.

---

Therapy is a learning process. Yet the person-centred therapist rarely if ever takes on the role of a teacher. Some clients seem to want or need to understand their own processing. Others do not. This may be a cultural or intellectual issue, or it may be that part of my trust in my client is to accord her the freedom to know or not know her processing.

I experience some clients as developing a keen sense of where in the room they want to focus their attention. Over a short period of time, a client may want first that I should understand how she feels, and then later will be concerned that I should be quiet so that she can think and feel about her own processing. What is it like for me? What happens to me? How do I do this? Can I do it differently?

In a nutshell, the most important skill in process work is to know when the client is engaged with her own process. For me to barge in upon this would be anti-therapeutic.

I conjecture that the learning process I refer to above is a dialogue between two puzzled people. The therapist is able to be aware of the client's processing, and to decide when to focus on this. The therapist is under no obligation to get it right on all occasions, but it is a good idea to talk about times when it feels wrong or awkward. The client becomes more able to internalize this therapeutic process and so will be able to live without therapy, moving fluently between spontaneous and reflexive living.

Andy helped me understand how a client could be both more spontaneous and more accurately reflexive at the same time.

---

**Case 3.2  Andy**

Andy, whom I have known for nearly two years, is talking about a new sense he has that he has a self which can exist, and is stable. 'I feel that I am no longer dirty. I am real. I don't have to think all the time that other people will find out how despicable I am. I can even stand up to my younger brother – well, sometimes.'

He seems to tell me this with surprised delight! He is animated. He looks me in the eye. He talks of his mother, who sexually abused him over some three years until he was taken into care, and does so with patent rage – out/rage. His body is alive with anger. It is still a struggle for me to come anywhere near to deep empathy with this experience. 'It has damaged me as a man', he said often enough. But I can draw near to his pain. But now, so different. Fluent – one of my favourite words of clients. Fluency is about having found some wholeness along the way.

'I know the memories still sear into you. I know how you must hate her. I can feel something of your anger as I listen, and I want to say, it feels good to hear it, as well as painful. I can still picture you with your hands hidden behind your back in those early sessions, like you dare not let them be seen to show what they felt. I really admire the flow of your anger.'

Maybe I don't say it quite like that. I spread out my empathic responding and my observing over time, but this summary will do.

---

## Reflection

As a therapist, I feel that I am able to be in touch with my client's process, responding to it. I enjoy what is healing. I am directed by his processing. I accept his new experience just as I did the old. (Healthy experiencing can be frightening to some clients.) I am actively and congruently in touch with his process in a way that embodies the core conditions.

In Andy's case, his process includes all those aspects of his experience, whether in or out of his awareness, that do not comprise the content or feelings of his story. His process includes his delight and all the signs which tell me that this is how he feels, his anger and all of the mental and physical aspects of this.

It includes the way and mood of his talking, the sensations within his body, the way he interacts with me, his use of his hands now to express rather than conceal feeling. His process also involves those changes indicated by his reworking of his story. His telling includes his anger. He becomes freely angry in the act of forth-telling. Underneath this, I suspect, is a changing self-concept. The meaning of the story changes because the meaning of Andy changes. He is no longer constricted by his past but can symbolize its pain as allowed and accepted anger.

Process can range from a single gesture to a new conception of a whole life story. It is about both the conscious and the unconscious material of the client and the therapist. As such it was inherent in Rogers' thinking from 1957 onwards (Frankel and Sommerbeck, 2007).

## 'A Process Conception of Psychotherapy'

Rogers' (1957c) paper is a watershed in more senses than one. It is, I contend, a loss of innocence for the person-centred movement. If there was ever a time when all that there was to person-centred therapy was a non-directive engagement with the client's conscious material, then it ended with this paper.

Carl Rogers' purpose was to seek to understand the process by which the client changed. His paper is a detailed phenomenological account of this process as he saw and had experienced it over 25 years of psychotherapy. The paper postulates two sets of elements to the process. The first is that the quality of client process changes in seven stages. The second is that there are a number of themes to this process. I cite Rogers' own words to describe these, using the seventh stage, although any of the stages would do just as well (Rogers, 1957c):

---

**Box 3.4  Rogers' descriptors of the seventh stage of psychotherapy**

New feelings are experienced with immediacy and richness of detail, both in the therapeutic relationship and outside. The experiencing of such feelings is used as a clear referent. There is a growing and continuing sense of acceptant ownership of these changing feelings, a basic trust in his own process.

Experiencing has lost almost completely its structure-bound aspects and becomes process experiencing – that is, the situation is experienced and interpreted in its newness, not as the past. The self becomes increasingly simply the subjective and reflexive awareness of experiencing. The self is much less frequently a perceived object, and much more frequently something confidently felt in process.

■ Personal constructs are tentatively reformulated, to be validated against further experience, but even then to be held loosely.

■ Internal communication is clear, with feelings and symbols well matched and fresh terms for new feelings. There is the experiencing of effective choice of new ways of being.

All knowledge is the end of innocence. Once I know that a client moves forward in therapy in the way described above, then I am more aware of the client as a whole human being. Of course, what Rogers writes is a series of generalizations, but in knowing these I, the therapist, am alerted to my client in new ways. There is no way back to a day when I did not know how my client's process changed with time.

All that is left to me is to decide how I may respond to this knowledge.

When I no longer believe that to engage with my client's process is essentially a contravention of the core conditions of therapy, when I see it as a deep relational possibility, I am faced with a choice that is inescapable in each and every moment of therapy.

Farber *et al.*'s (1996) *The Psychotherapy of Carl Rogers: Cases and Commentary* offers a magisterial insight into Rogers' own practice. The commentaries represent the literalist and the experientialist perspectives, as well as the views of psychodynamically orientated practitioners. One of the major controversies embodied here concerns the argument put forward by Maria Villas-Boas Bowen that Rogers' principles had remained constant but his practice had changed between the 'non-directive' early phase and his mature work. I end this chapter with her summary of her own observations. It seems to me that if she is correct then Rogers is engaging in process work in a way that is congruent with my own standpoint:

> Forty-five years later, we hear him verbalizing attitudes that the client has not yet introduced, offering and testing interpretations, and often being quite directive with the client. I think the biggest change of all is that he trusted his clients more. He considered them to be less fragile and less easily damageable by comments made by the therapist. He was more trusting of the client's self-determination and self-regulation and saw his clients as less at the mercy of the therapist's influence. This gave him, I believe, more flexibility, freedom and congruence with the kind of person he had become. But one thing he never changed was his belief in the core values underlying his work in psychotherapy.
>
> (M. Villas-Boas Bowen, 'The Case of Jill: Commentary' in
> Farber *et al.*, 1996, p. 94)

In the following two sections of this book, engaging with client process will be seen in terms of an understanding first of phenomenology and then of existentialism. In Chapter 13, engaging with Hilary's process will exemplify this potential, alongside one fascinating paradigm of the client's process by which to understand Hilary further.

# Further Reading

Barrett-Lennard, G.T. (1998) *Carl Rogers' Helping System: Journey and substance.* London: Sage.

  This is the most authoritative of overviews of Rogers' work, combining history, biography and theoretical development. It is the key text for understanding how Rogers' thought comes together. Of particular use are chapters 6, 12 and 13 in thinking about process.

Rennie, D. (1998) *Person-Centred Counselling: An Experiential Approach.* London, Sage.

  Chapter seven of this book gives an accessible account of process direction. It is also one of the sources of my thinking on spontaneous and reflexive processing. Chapter eight on metacommunication is, I think, essential reading for those of all approaches who wish to be congruent with their clients.

Villas-Boas Bowen, M. (1996) 'The Myth of Non-Directiveness: The case of Jill'. In Farber *et al.* (1996), pp. 74–94.

  A thoroughly worked-through argument that non-directivity is less central to person-centred therapy than others would have us believe. It, like all of the case studies in this volume, gives huge insight into the practice of therapy. It needs to be read alongside the paper to which it acts as a counter-claim, Grant (1990).

# Part II
## Phenomenological Perspectives

# 4

# A Phenomenological
# Approach to Therapy

The first three chapters have set out an argument that process work is an integral aspect of addressing the client's frame of reference. It is therefore a necessary aspect of any holistic, phenomenological therapy.

In this chapter, the concept of phenomenology is introduced and explained. The case of Lesley illustrates how forgetting the principles of phenomenology can lead the therapist to misjudge the nature and contents of the client's frame of reference. This is related to process work through three practical principles derived from Spinelli's description of phenomenology. The case of Evelyn demonstrates that active process work involves the therapist in trusting more fully the client's process and hence the client herself. Lastly, a phenomenological approach to therapy is linked to theory integration.

Rennie's work with process identification is described. I see it as superficial and tool-like. Process work is closer to depth reflection, a form of empathy. These accounts of the relationship between phenomenological principles and the therapist's understanding of the client's frame of reference lead to a number of practical guidelines. However, an understanding of the principles of phenomenology also open up the possibility of person-centred practice as integrative, and this is explored at the end of this chapter, with particular reference to Chapters 6 and 7.

We begin the exploration with the case of Lesley, in which much learning came from my getting it wrong for her.

---

**Case 4.1   Lesley**

When I met Lesley, she was a 32-year old shop assistant, fairly recently married to Vyvyan. At 15, she had gone out with an older man – some ten years her senior – against her mother's wishes. He raped her. Mother had consistently punished her for her 'disobedience'. Mother was cold and withholding. (Emotional warmth

---

could only be given as a reward for her children being as she needed them to be.)

Lesley had been taken to the doctor for a pregnancy test, but under strictest instructions not to reveal the assault. That was her disgrace and she would have to learn to live with it. After the test, which proved negative, there came silence. Lesley lived, she felt, with the constant underlying message that she was not to be trusted with men. Her adolescence was, on the surface, painfully conservative from then on. She met Vyvyan when she was 25. Two years later they planned to marry. Half way through this period of preparation for the wedding, Lesley became pregnant. She took herself off and had an abortion without Vyvyan knowing.

Lesley had been able to tell Vyvyan about the rape before they married. It had some effect upon her sexual feelings and responses, but less than she had feared. He was patient and understanding, and at first the love, security and even maternal approval of marriage helped her relax.

However, there was the constant but unconscious presence of Mother's cold and scolding voice: 'You can't be trusted with men.' It was not clear to me whether the message – 'And so you cannot trust them either' – came from Lesley's experience or her mother's 'voice'.

Lesley came to therapy because the injunction to feel untrustworthy came to the fore when Vyvyan broached the subject of having a child of their own. She experienced panic at the thought of parenthood. There were occasional bouts of vaginismus if she felt unsafe about her contraception. There was guilt about the abortion and occasional flashbacks to the rape.

In the early part of therapy, Lesley worked with the fear of being a parent. There gradually emerged a sense that her concept of herself-as-mother was modelled upon the punitive coldness of her own mother. Who else could have killed their own child? (It struck me that her own mother had indeed come close to a psychic killing of Lesley.) For weeks these sessions were interspersed with fleeting and then more complete recall of her rape. There was a battle within her about how trustworthy I was. This, I felt – but never reflected to her – was not just as a man, one with the form, the shape of a rapist, but because she was able to project her lack of faith in herself onto me, and work with it within the confines of a hopefully trustworthy and real relationship. We also spent the last 15 minutes of about five sessions on basic relaxation exercises to counter the panic. This was clearly negotiated and seemingly effective as a way of learning to cope with an unpleasant symptom.

By session 16, Lesley had begun to formulate the idea of her mother's voice in her head. For two sessions, I listened carefully as Lesley began to hear, as if for the first time, that so much of what she felt about herself came from Mother. At the end of session 17, she expressed genuine gratitude and surprise that at last a human being had heard her with understanding. It was not about rape but about being radically untrustworthy. My own reaction to this was that it felt as though she had heard herself for the first time. The gratitude was also a projection. It was genuine too. I much enjoyed it. Unfortunately I was hooked by it, and jumped the gun.

In session 18, Lesley began to reflect that she had experienced over the week a freeing up of her view of herself. I responded that she now felt, I guess, that she had more of a choice about how she saw herself, and how she could picture Vyvyan's love for her – more real now. She acknowledged this warmly as part of her thinking and feeling. 'Now I can hear Mother more clearly I can decide whether I like what she says to me, whether it fits.' Buoyed up by 'my success' – and how toxic that is for therapists! – and her real pleasure and relief, Richard-the-Rescuer took empathy one stage too far: 'And I guess you have more freedom to choose about a baby now.'

Achievement gave way in Lesley to tears of anger. I had intruded. She thought I had understood.

The next session was a time of repair and painful honesty. I had simply jumped the gun. 'I was OK, because its OK to get it wrong.' But underneath I felt nothing of the sort, for a while.

## Reflection

My intervention was way off mark. The motivation for it was, I am sure, a careless desire to short-cut the client's process. 'All this is true for you, so I guess that having a baby might be easier too.' It all seems quite crass when I look back. I was outside of my client's frame of reference – not with her. What follows aims to develop a feel for what it can mean to be outside of another's frame of reference.

Mearns and Thorne (1999, p. 46) put forward a useful and simple empathy scale. The fourth level is described thus:

This response shows an understanding of the client beyond the level of the client's immediate awareness. As well as communicating comprehension of the surface feelings and responses of the client, the listener is showing an understanding of *underlying* feelings. This is sometimes called 'additive empathy', but is more commonly referred to as *depth reflection*.

(Original emphases)

I know the value of being in touch with the deeper elements of the client's feelings. This part of her frame of reference can be available to the therapist even when it is out of the client's immediate awareness. Depth reflection can be crucial in the relationship with the client. It is also open to carelessness or even abuse. I was careless because I did not check out that my so-called 'intuition' was actually part of the client's way of seeing the world. I was falling short of the phenomenological method.

There is a fine line between empathy on the one hand and speculation on the other. Speculation can be useful in person-centred therapy in the sense of being puzzled with the client. It must be owned as such, openly. What I had done was to extend the *cognitive logic* of where the client was, and applied it to the core presenting problem. The client was not yet there. Clients' processes within themselves are a complex mixture of thinking, feeling and other types of self-experiencing. They are simply not open to the kind of logic I was applying.

Lesley had reached a point whereby she could talk of her mother as the origin of many of her fears and self-condemnations. She could hear her mother's voice more clearly, and come to make decisions. There had been in three or so sessions of therapy a shift in her self-concept. For her this had been incorporated into her thinking; it was a cognitive as well as an affective shift. She felt different but also understood differently. When in Chapter 13 we look at Greenberg *et al.*'s (1993) understanding of the human mind, we will see that they put forward a clear but complex relationship between affect, emotion and cognition which suggests that cognition usually follows emotion – the exact opposite of the cognitive therapist's view that emotion follows understanding (Weishaar, 1993, p. 48). It seems to me that my client was processing at a number of levels, some of the material out of her awareness and some within it. At the first level she was noting how it felt to recognize mother's voice for what it was. At the second level, she was utilizing these feelings to extend her self-understanding in cognitive and emotional domains of her self-concept. The third level is the transferential level, which I will discuss below.

My error was to jump the gun as far as her own processing was concerned. She had not yet made the links between her recognizing her mother's toxic voice and her struggle to trust herself and Vyvyan to conceive a child. These links I had treated as logical and rational. They are not. They are emotional and affective links. The process of recognizing a new resource is like the seeping of a warm liquid into parched tissue. It takes time. It can be resisted. I tried to hurry it. I was outside of Lesley's frame of reference just because I forgot to listen to her gradual change in self-valuing. Frame of reference is a complex notion, intimately linked with the client's *way* of processing.

My error was experienced as an unbearable intrusion. In leaving Lesley's frame of reference I had triggered a transferential relationship. Transference is the phenomenon whereby people treat one person *as if* they were someone else, someone who is either seen as powerfully positive or powerfully negative. Thus, for some while I had become her mother – 'You must *seem* OK even if you can't be trusted'. I could have responded to this disastrously, by obliging my client's projection and becoming her mother for her – cold and punishing – while experiencing myself as hurt, withdrawn and self-punishing. This process is called projective identification – a sort of unconscious giving in to the transference or projected feelings (Klein 1988a,b; Segal, 1992). Fortunately, I had the opportunity to own my self-acceptance even when in error, and so be congruently Richard in the face of the transference. This moving through the transference to a genuine relationship is characteristically person-centred (Rogers, 1951, pp. 198–218), although I note that some psychodynamic therapists take a similar line (for instance, Guntrip, 1992).

I left my client's frame of reference because I lost for a moment or two a grasp of how she was processing understanding against affect, and that largely out of her awareness.

## Frame of Reference as a Phenomenological Concept

Being person-centred needs to be rooted in the therapist's conscious understanding of the principles of phenomenology. I set out in the following sections the key themes.

Phenomenology is a study or theory of human knowledge. How and what do we know? How do we know what we know and how do we know it is true? Phenomenology teaches us to listen in a new way to people, because it underpins this listening with a humility about what the client and the therapist can possibly know of each other. We learn to listen with new ears. I suggest that I was not listening in this way to Lesley, albeit for a few moments only.

The question of knowing has a very long history indeed. The common-or-garden answer today is the modernist one that the securest form of knowledge is scientific knowledge. Even though this would seem strange to most of humanity throughout history, popular scientific culture maintains the myth that knowledge is objective. It is 'out there' and is not particularly disturbed by the knower.

In fact, science proper has not been like this since the end of the nineteenth century. Relativity theory and quantum mechanics thoroughly undermined the notion that science was like a common-sense understanding of how a machine worked. The physical world at either very small scale or very high energy behaves in ways that can only be described with difficulty. Common sense no longer tells us the objective truth even about the physical world. Thomas Kuhn (1962) systematically laid to rest the myth that science works by being

objective. His influential argument was that scientists think in very conservative ways – on tramlines called paradigms. It takes an intellectual earthquake to
bring about a paradigm shift. Far from being objective, science can be bound
by the fear of new ways of thinking.

Humanistic psychology has its own paradigm, its own characteristic way
of thinking (Spinelli, 1989; McLeod, 1996). It is a paradigm which sets its
face against the mythical primacy of objective knowledge. Knowing is also
subjective – deeply part of the shared encounter of all human beings from
within their self-experiencing.

## Phenomenology and Practice

The twentieth-century German philosopher, Edmund Husserl, developed
modern phenomenology. Although his work is complex, the key ideas behind
it are not. They invite us to see our knowing about the world in a very different
light. He argued that we must give up the illusion that we can know objec-
tively about things and people. The problem with knowledge is that we only
see through our *own* eyes. The very act of seeing, hearing, understanding is
already an interpretation by us. The truth does not come to us uncontaminated
by who we are.

Empathy is the act of understanding how others assemble themselves.
I remember a client who was forbidden anger; when she felt angry she would
describe her feelings as 'a bit cross'. This language stood for the incongruity
between her affect and her socially constructed way of expressing and experiencing anger. As we worked on the language, the feelings gradually came. Both
empathy and congruence are rooted in the fact that we put together our own
world in the complexities of our subjective experience. There may be truth out
there – or not, as the case may be – but we cannot receive it immediately. Like
an old radio set, there is always interference. The phenomenological method
aims to acknowledge this fully and to work with the interference.

As I listened to Lesley, I jumped to a wrong conclusion: if she could see
most of her life differently now, then she should surely be able to see all of it in
that way, including having a baby. Had I been alert to the phenomenological
perspective, then I would have recognized that she was not processing in that
way. The cognitive penny had dropped, but the working through at the emotional level was to take some weeks. The self-concept is 'modular'. Human
beings change their self-structure area by area, and not as a whole.

Every act of perceiving is a distorting of what is there. This sounds like common sense, but we miss how radical it is. As I look at the paper in the computer
printer now, I see that it is darker than the paper lying flat on the desk. This
does not worry me. I know that the light is falling differently on it. I instinc-
tively bracket out this difference as irrelevant. As I make myself aware of it,
I see the distorting effect of different light sources, but until I reflect deeply

I do not notice or perhaps even fully know about the distortion that comes from my spectacle lenses, from the shape of my eyeball – I am myopic – from the acuity of my optic nerve, from the sight centres of my brain, and ultimately from my higher functions of awareness within the cerebral neo-cortex. Society tells me how to see paper. It is white – but is it? It is blank, but I only think this because I know what writing is. Even the paper in my printer is a social construct. My deviant senses are not as trustworthy as I presume. What am I to do?

The first step for the therapist, I suggest, is to know that the person-centred approach is not a mere option. It is founded upon a radical theory of knowledge. It is not possible for me to know another person 'directly'. Now I see through a glass darkly. To be person-centred is to assert firmly that our knowledge is more limited than we care to admit. Whenever I am tempted to move away from the phenomenological perspective I need to be aware of how much I think, erroneously, I can know about the client.

---

**Box 4.1    Spinelli's three principles**

Ernesto Spinelli puts forward three actions which are necessary to listening accurately. These he derives from the philosophy of Edmund Husserl:

- Bracket off your preconceptions and prejudices by first becoming as fully aware of them as you can, and then set them aside. Know that you will not succeed fully.
- Never explain or interpret. Only describe. Even accurate description is difficult. It is in explanation that we bring to bear our own characteristic distortions of others' material.
- Horizontalize. Give equal weight to each aspect of what is being described.

---

The phenomenological method then puts forward a number of practical manoeuvres which I can make in order to exercise my responsibility as a listener. Ernesto Spinelli (1989/2005) summarizes these as three steps (Spinelli, 1989, pp. 17–9). The first of these is epoche, or bracketing. It is not possible to be free of bias, but we can be more effective when we bracket off our prejudices. This is an act of self-awareness, and underlines the primacy of personal development in the therapist's life. Prejudice here has a range of meanings. It can be prejudice in the sense that it is acted out towards those of other race, ability, gender or sexual orientation. It also, for instance, involves the bias of not-seeing. Thus I did not see that Lesley had not completed a set of affective processes. I 'chose' not to, but was unaware of my choice. Bracketing can never be known to be fully effective. It rarely is. It is better to have tried and lost than never to have tried at all. Phenomenology teaches us the depth of care, even caution, we need in the allegedly simple act of empathizing.

The second step Spinelli terms the rule of description. Never explain or interpret, only describe. This distinction is subtle. It includes a renouncing of interpretation in the psychodynamic sense of the word: 'This is the meaning of what you have experienced.' But it is more about an attitude than what is done on any occasion. Identical words can be said to a client with two underlying attitudes: *You're feeling the sadness of it all. I sort of see it in your eyes.* Some therapists can offer an apparently empathic comment with the air of a diagnosis. Some clients have been all too used to being told what to feel, and they will oblige. If the underlying attitude is, 'I see what is going on', then the phenomenological awareness of the therapist is not adequately tuned in. The alternative attitude is that the observation hovers as a question. As Carl Rogers expressed it:

> Each response of mine contains the unspoken question, 'Is this the way it is for you? Am I catching just the color and texture and flavor of the personal meaning you are experiencing just now? If not, I wish to bring my perception in line with yours.'
> (Rogers, 1986b, in Kirschenbaum and Henderson, 1990a, p. 128)

The added reference to physical process – sadness in the eyes – is offered in the same way as evidence, but always open to contradiction, for I can only describe, not assign meaning. It is important in work with clients and groups to foster an air of uncertainty of meaning or accuracy in the therapist. There is a delicate balance between alleged empathy that is overmuch sure of itself and that which is irritatingly insecure. Be in touch with your client, but be prepared to ask, to stop, to check.

The third step is the rule of horizontalization. Give every utterance of the client equal value. It is important to note the distortions that can occur when we paraphrase. I reflected this but not that. Why? One reason might be that I could not bear to notice my client's grief because I am grieving myself. However, another reason might be that one particular part of what my client said stands out for me. I choose, consciously or otherwise, to focus. This can be a conscious helping of the client to focus, in accordance with their own expressed wish – and that is not controversial. I do note that much of my own focusing is about therapeutic awareness within me. If the client offers me an apparently neutral comment followed by a comment that strongly suggests a condition of worth in operation – an ought – I will opt to focus on the latter. To do so is therapeutic. In practice, there is considerable difference in degrees of horizontalizing between one therapist and another. The phenomenological commitment is to be aware.

The practical guidelines of phenomenological method are based upon a number of abstract principles. These can be informative of our counselling too.

Franz Brentano, the Viennese philosopher who taught Husserl, developed the word 'intentionality' to describe a very particular attribute of the human mind (Spinelli, 1989; Moustakas, 1994). It has nothing to do with the usual meaning of the word 'intention'. It is from the Latin verb *intendere* – to stretch forth. It refers to a stretching forth of the mind to the phenomena of the outside world. The human mind is always processing, interpreting the raw data of experience. What we call our experience is already interpreted. We cannot get to the Thing-Itself of experience.

It is at precisely this point I believe the classical approach can be misguided; it speaks of tracking the client with a knowledge that only the client is an expert on themselves. Of course, I wholly agree that the therapist cannot be an expert on the client. How could she be? The client's material is just not available to the therapist in that way. Phenomenology teaches us to be humble about what we can possibly know. Being person-centred is a commitment to a theory of knowledge as well as a way of being. Person-Centred therapists have no neutral territory from which to judge others' material. *To the extent that the client is also limited by the way of knowing, it is surely the case that the client also has no privileged access to her own awareness.* I object to the notion that clients are experts on themselves.

---

**Box 4.2  Comparing frames of reference**

I am grateful to a supervisee of mine, Liz Orrell, who put this in a really useful illustration for me. I say, I have an apple. You say, I too have an apple. We compare what we perceive. I have a pear and you a lemon. We think: That does not fit. In other words, truth comes at times in a relationship from the comparing of the frames of reference of two puzzled individuals. I suggest that this congruent activity is especially characteristic of the later parts of the counselling relationship when trust is secure. It is also far more appropriate with some clients than others – and that depends on how the client tends to process their own awareness.

---

By way of illustration, let us return to Lesley's introject: 'You cannot be trusted with men'. At first, I had no understanding of this, no way of knowing where this came from, what it was, what it felt like, how it really impacted upon Lesley's life. Likewise, Lesley had already interpreted her mother's message as if it were a fact-out-there. It is really the case that I cannot be trusted with men. She then proceeded to reframe all of her available evidence to match this.

Neither she nor I were experts in her material. New light dawns from the space between us, from Rogers' mutual act of striving to understand (Ogden, 1992). This phenomenological perspective will allow us to see afresh the purposes of working with the client at the level of her process as well as her content and feelings.

## The 'What' and 'How' of Experiencing

Husserl distinguished two aspects of any knowing: the *noema* and the *noesis*. The *noematic* focus of experience is the object-as-perceived – the 'what'? of our experiencing. The *noetic* focus is the way, the category of our perceiving – the 'how'? of our experiencing. This is not an easy distinction to make. It is difficult because we do not normally recognize the limits of our knowing in this way. An example may help. As I write, I am looking out of the window at a tree in the car park of the school opposite my house. I notice that it is a curious and irregular shape. The top seems a little off-set, while the left-hand side of it in silhouette is ragged and tooth-like. To the right, it descends swiftly for a while and then forms a bulb of leaves and branches – smoother, rounder. The right side is greener, lighter in colour.

The first recognition that I make is that this is not the Tree-Itself. There really is a tree, of course, but it is a transcendental object. That is to say, it always goes beyond our possible experiencing. The subjective myth is that I experience the tree. I do not. I experience my experiencing of the tree. The modernist scientific myth is that I can encapsulate the objective essence of the tree descriptively and quantitatively. I cannot. The modernist myth simply causes me not to notice what I cannot encapsulate. The tree is 'out there', but my experience is within me. There is a version of the tree within me, but it is only a version.

What I experience, and habitually but wrongly call the tree, has two foci. The *noematic* focus is made up of the experience of the data which come from the tree. I perceive its shape, but that is governed by where I am. If I move, it has a different shape. The *noetic* focus is the aspect of my experiencing by which I put the tree together. Therefore I note that I call the round shape to the right, bulbous. The metaphor is from within me, and not from the tree. I call the lighter colour 'more green', but I note that others could just as legitimately call the darker portions 'more green'. The *noema* of the tree flows to me from the Tree-Itself that I cannot perceive. The *noesis* comes from my ways of perceiving, my habits, my categories.

Note that this feels difficult. It is not just that we do not habitually think in this way. It is also that the *noema* and *noesis* are two foci of the same experiencing. They cannot be separated. I cannot know for sure which is which. I could not bracket off one of these foci. They are in perpetual tension and interpenetration.

The distinction between the *noema* and the *noesis* of experiencing is all-important, for it teaches us to note that all experience is both received and constructed. Whatever I experience is not only different from the Thing-Itself, the transcendental object, but is also made up of a weave of the so-called 'raw data', or rather raw-data-as-I-experience-it and my way of assembling that both cognitively and emotionally. This weave is tight; the weft and warp cannot be disentangled. To experience is both to receive and construct. It happens seamlessly. Why does this matter?

All experiencing is a combination of the imperfect and selective act of perceiving together with the act of interpreting in terms of categories open to the individual. Let us call this combination a process. Each person processes differently. Therefore, in order to empathize, I must have some idea of how my processing connects with my client's processing.

From a phenomenological perspective, process involves a sort of dialogue between the 'what' of subjective perceiving and the 'how' of perceiving. The 'how' is determined by the whole mental apparatus of the subject. The 'how' of perceiving relates closely to the self-concept. Thus, the person who has experienced many conditions of worth will perceive with a suspicion or even with built-in self-condemnation verging on paranoia.

# Anger

The best way I know of to explore the truth of the rich diversity of 'how'? and 'what'? in our experiencing is to talk with a number of friends and relatives about their experience of anger. Try this as phenomenological research in miniature.

What does the other person notice about someone who is angry with them? What do they notice about their reactions? How do they feel? What do they do? What do they believe they are required to do, if anything? Do they avoid anger or engage with it? Is getting angry good or bad? Is it normally their fault or the other person's fault if they get angry with them? Do they feel that they can *make* others angry, or does the other person choose? Do others *make* them angry, or do they choose anger?

This research is likely to give you a sense that people put anger together in radically different ways. This relates to the role of anger – or fantasies of anger – in embedding conditions of worth in our self-concept. Anger in ourselves and others is a potent psychological experience in earliest life and in the present. You will have noticed that you are not exempt from this messy process. Like me, you will put anger together in your own characteristic way.

In counsellor education, congruence often develops as the ability to face anger in others and oneself. Sometimes that is real anger, sometimes imagined or projected. Occasionally we experience anger because of projective identification. Others 'cause' us unconsciously to experience anger 'for' them.

Sometimes students feel angry with tutors transferentially. It is about imagined power and its abuse. Sometimes this is real enough. The tutor got it wrong, even abusively.

To engage empathically with another human being, particularly in those psychologically significant categories like anger, is to need to be in touch with the way that person processes. This can be seen in the case of Evelyn.

---

**Case 4.2 Evelyn**

Evelyn is married to Gerald, a psychotherapist, who, for reasons I am not yet quite sure of, is unable to engage with his own emotions and hence hers (or is it the other way round?). She does not describe herself as unhappily married, but she is clearly not emotionally fulfilled. She is largely silent about Gerald to date.

She was, until six months ago, the deputy head of a large comprehensive school. Falling rolls, personal and professional issues, and reorganization at school had led to her redundancy and much acrimony. She came to see me, presenting as rejected and depressed. Above all, she felt a strong but futile (her construct) anger towards her head teacher and the deputy chair of the school's governing body. Anger was futile, she believed, because any expression of it would compromise her future career. I noted within me the probability that this was a rationalization, a defence against her deeper anger.

In talking with Evelyn, I noted how her severe and yet precise and caring exterior seemed to remain largely unemotional. No tears, little apparent stress, but resigned, constricted, held in.

The legal process of her redundancy was coming to an end. After a while, there came a strange, almost peaceful equilibrium. She no longer turned her anger against herself as she had once done. Yet she had seemingly renounced outward rage as 'unwise'.

I had noted from the first sessions of our work that Evelyn did not easily talk about her feelings. A question like 'What are you feeling now?' was doubly significant for me. In the early days of a relationship, I tend to go with Pete Sanders' dictum that questions even about feelings are interruptive, perhaps directive (Frankland and Sanders, 1995, p. 123). The fact that I asked the question told me that I felt distanced from her feeling-process and was objecting to this within myself. The question would produce a long silence – two or three minutes. I felt ever more irritated, distanced, puzzled. Yet the question also emphasized Evelyn's presenting of herself in our second session as someone with a large gap between her head and her heart, her thinking and feeling processes.

I reflected her process to her: I notice that you pause for a long while when you are trying to get in touch with what you feel. Evelyn explained that she was trying to escape into her head. Yet, this calm explanation for my sake did not seem to ring true. Defences, I felt, are rarely so obliging as to present themselves thus:

R: So what are you doing now?
E: Consulting.
R: What are you feeling?
E: Scared.
R: I'm wondering where do you feel that, if that makes sense to you.
E: I understand what you mean, but (Another long pause) I don't know.
R: It is as if you *experience* emotion but don't know where or how you can check it out?
E: That's it.

I felt within me a desire somehow to get stuck in and get Evelyn in touch with her emotion. That must surely be the way forward. Fortunately I had the good sense to do nothing of the sort.

I remained with the 'gap between head and heart' for a number of sessions. It dawned upon me only gradually that, far from wanting to 'correct' Evelyn's processing, I had come to trust it. She would still take long pauses. She would consult inwardly. Still the long silence could feel frustrating, but I noted that her answers to the silence, the fruits of her consulting, were becoming very reliable. I did not need to interfere to correct any process. In spite of my irritation with waiting upon her, she did seem after all to have a fair idea of what she felt, even if she did not know where that answer was coming from. Moreover, I no longer needed to ask. She would consult increasingly of her own volition, and that felt good.

Several sessions later, I again reflected to Evelyn her process of pausing to consult inwardly. This time I added that I had come to trust it. It seemed to me to work. I added that it was as if she could know her feelings but was not allowed to feel them. Like not being allowed to *ask* for what you want?

Evelyn paused. With clarity that I found moving, she responded, *I wasn't allowed to want.*

## Reflection

How can I not want what I want? It must be that I do not feel what I feel. Many clients will deny their feelings as unacceptable. Evelyn fought hard to discover hers. They were powerful, strong and felt dangerous. But they had no 'place' in her. She looked and found the answer, but did not find out where she was looking. It has subsequently emerged that Evelyn has within her two sub-systems: one contains her organismic needs, while the other disapproves fearfully. The latter resolutely declined to 'look inside' the former, but Evelyn's cognitive overview of her Self had not repressed her awareness of her emotions.

I now see this state of affairs as the product of years of processing. One part of her desperately wants to know her feelings; and she can access them powerfully, even fearfully. Yet, the very feelings which, I guess, she has learned to access are still denied symbolization in her body. This contrasts with the state of affairs described by Rogers (1957c) in which the fully functioning client has 'feelings and symbols well matched, and fresh terms for new feelings' (Rogers, 1957c, p. 154). Evelyn can know what she feels but not locate this somatically. It is not a flight into the head, but fully felt emotion deprived of its quality of desire. She is not allowed to want.

I am struck by three movements in this piece of work with Evelyn. The first concerns frustration; the second, understanding; the third, progress, revelation, a leap of awareness.

Evelyn had felt herself to be stuck in her head. This was frustrating. The time it took her to consult herself was also a sharing of frustration. Her sense of being kept out of touch with the very feelings she experienced so strongly needed to be communicated to me. My empathic desire to understand her process was also the vehicle for my introjecting her frustration as if it were mine. Had I over-identified and taken it to be mine, I would have lost touch with her experiencing. In order to remain in contact with her deeper experience – as opposed to her declared feeling – I had to remain with that process, the silence, searching and hesitation. Had I interfered, interpreted or tried to overcome the apparent resistance, then the moment would have been lost.

Understanding came from an intuition on my part that her process, far from being as unreliable as she thought, was indeed a useful if unusual way of accessing feeling. I came to see this in the normal run of therapy. It was a while before it occurred to me that Evelyn could access her feelings strongly and feel their threat.

In looking actively with Evelyn at her processing, I was able to affirm my trust in it. I then offered a fairly unimaginative empathic response: able but not permitted to feel feelings. I tried to embody in this something of a paradox, or perhaps just my own confusion. There lurked here Rogers' concealed question: am I anywhere near how it is? Evelyn then pointed to the act of wanting as the forbidden to her.

## Process Work: Theory and Practice

David Rennie (1998) has given a number of valuable examples of what he terms process identification (both historical and present), process direction and metacommunication (Rennie, 1998, chapters seven and eight). By process identification, he means an active noticing of the client's process; by direction, he means a brief suggestion as to what the client might choose to do; by metacommunication, he means second-order speech about the quality of communication that is going on between client and therapist. The last of these is similar to Gerard Egan's immediacy skills (Egan, 1990, pp. 224–9). The ways of intervening to which Rennie points are useful, if used in a person-centred way. My argument with Rennie, as I have previously said, is to do with his language of therapist expertise concerning the client's process.

Of course, all person-centred therapists aim for expertise in being person-centred. If they do not, they leave themselves open to complaint and litigation. However, Rennie positions his approach as midway between the purist approach and the holistic but directive approach of Gendlin. The latter he describes as 'directive in terms of the client's process and non-directive in terms of the client's content' (Rennie, 1998, p. 2). His own approach 'entails counsellor directiveness of the client's processing of experience when it seems warranted by both client and counsellor' (Rennie, 1998, p. 1).

He gives the following example of a dialogue illustrating therapist direction of the client's process (Rennie, 1998, p. 82):

---

**Box 4.3   Process direction**

*Counsellor*: You're remembering feeling like crying, but can't seem to take it further than that.
*Client*: Yeah. I don't know why. Like – I don't – I don't – I don't know. Like this morning I was putting my make-up on and I started crying.
*Counsellor*: It seems like both the source and the nature of your feelings are unclear. I'm wondering if it might be useful to concentrate on those feelings to see if something comes up.

---

I note that this last intervention is directive, but is easily containable within a person-centred relationship. It presumes – at least in my practice – that the foundation of trust is already in place; that there is full and mutual permission for such a miniature experiment, and that it is part of a larger process of tracking the client, rather than of taking charge of the session. I also note that some person-centred therapists would be more at ease with this than others. That is fine!

My contention here is that Rennie does not pay sufficient, sustained attention to the nature of process, and is therefore more concerned with the surface
activity of the therapist, and less with work in depth. I contrast this with
the work of Mearns who seems to me to have a far firmer grasp of process
in his work with his client Elizabeth, while remaining firmly committed to
the necessity and sufficiency of the core conditions (Mearns, 1994a; Mearns,
1994b).

I have quoted Rennie's definition of process in Chapter 2. I note that it
consists largely of a string of gerunds, or verbal nouns. Process is what the
client *does*. This way of talking makes process accessible. I can see and notice
what people do. Yet process is reduced to client behaviour. The meanings
of this behaviour seem not to be as important to him. I suggest that client
process, and indeed process within the whole of the counselling relationship, is
not this simple. It must be seen from a phenomenological perspective. Process
is a deep, inward set of psychological events.

To see this, we return to Evelyn. She has been hurt and possibly abused in
a work situation. Let us call her basic experience rejection. (It is of course not
that simple in reality.) That experience has a *noematic* and a *noetic* focus. It has
a 'what'? and a 'how'? to it. What is true of a tree is even more clearly true of
'rejection'. She neither has a grasp of the Thing-Itself nor does she see at first
how she construes the experience for herself. The word 'rejection', unlike the
word 'tree', is itself value-laden. One person in a relationship can feel rejected
while the other person protests that this was not their intent.

I suggest that a simple description of Evelyn's experiencing and processing
would look like this, from her point of view. First, her job is at risk. She perceives a set of data that imply that at least. But do the data also imply that it
is *her* job because she is in some way unacceptable to the school, or her head
teacher or the governors? The basic data of redundancy is associated with other
data concerning non-acceptability. The *noematic* focus is full of ambivalences.
Do the other data-sets warrant the conclusion that Evelyn is in fact unacceptable to her school? Does the association of both sets of data hold water? This
is *noematic* to the extent that an outside observer with as full an access to facts
as possible might either be uncertain or agree with Evelyn that she is being
discriminated against, or might decide that Evelyn is showing signs of paranoia. In other words, the data, the raw facts, are already interpreted in the act
of perceiving and in the act of associating different perception-sets.

So far, the need to process information as knowledge has been seen solely
from a *noematic* perspective. Evelyn's *noetic* focus concerns, as far as I can
be aware at the moment, her condition of worth, namely, that she must not
want. When she is denied a natural need, like job satisfaction, employment
itself, approval for her work, then she both feels emotions and discounts them.
She is aware that she has an almost child-like sense of seeking affirmation,
even attention. Yet she has learned to perceive this internal message as dangerous, or at the very least not worth paying attention to. Whereas some clients

seem blissfully out of touch with their feelings, Evelyn avoids them because she knows them only too clearly, even if she can 'switch them off' on some occasions. However, together with these feelings goes a construction that it is wrong/dangerous/thankless to pay attention to them.

This processing goes on continuously within Evelyn. It is this processing which embodies the qualities such as awareness and symbolization to which Rogers (1957c) points. The external behaviour may be a clue to it. Phenomenologically, the therapist and client explore this together. It is difficult. The therapist is certainly not an expert on the client's process, although she may have knowledge of others' processing which may be useful or deceptive. The client is not always an expert. She too can be confused. However, the one difference – and this is the significant one for person-centred work – is that when the penny drops for the client, then there may well be a nascent accurate and incontrovertible insight. Only the client can have an incorrigible sense of insight.

The therapist and client alike listen to the client's process. Often, both are puzzled. Yet the therapist trusts this puzzling process. What Rennie calls process identification and direction should be little more than a specialized and immediate empathy, not with feelings but with process. The therapist seeks to wrestle with experiential and existential understanding, but only the client has the power to recognize.

To the client's process the therapist can then accord empathy – is this how you feel/see/do it? – and unconditional positive regard – there is no right way of processing, only what you freely decide.

In terms of counsellor congruence, there are two other interlinking and complex processes going on. First, just as the client processes in characteristic ways, so does the therapist. Both empathy and congruence require me as a therapist to understand something of my own processing. From time to time, I feel it right to say to a client: that is just not how I feel/see/do it. This is an invitation to work in terms of the difference between us, in just the same way that empathy is a wrestling with not understanding as well as understanding. Secondly, the relationship has a characteristic way of processing too. I experience my processing with each client as being different. If I respond intuitively to the client, I will adapt to them. At best this will be empathic adaptation, at worst, unhelpful counter-transference and defensiveness.

Process in counselling is deeper and more complex than David Rennie states or illustrates. A client's processing is part of her frame of reference. We are committed as best we can to track and reflect that too.

## Phenomenology and Integration

Understanding what is the client's phenomenology and being committed to her actualizing tendency are the two basic tenets of person-centred practice.

All else flows from this. I have argued above that the therapist's behaviour is a flexible response to these movements of understanding and trust, and are not set down on tablets of stone. However, the same is true of the use of theory. Much of what follows in this book is a reflection on theories, some from within and some from beyond person-centred thought. The last few years have seen a growth in the United Kingdom of an openness to other theory (Worsley, 2007a). How might this work in practice?

I want to return to part of my consideration of my work with Lesley (Case Study 4.1). I had leapt ahead of where Lesley really was. I wrote,

> My error was experienced as an unbearable intrusion. In leaving Lesley's frame of reference I had triggered a transferential relationship. For some while I had become her mother – 'You must *seem* OK even if you can't be trusted'. I could have responded to this disastrously, by obliging my client's projection and becoming her mother for her – cold and punishing – while experiencing myself as hurt, withdrawn and self-punishing. This process is called projective identification – a sort of unconscious giving in to the transference or projected feelings.

These minutes of therapy were traumatic for Lesley. She felt herself pushed back into old and disturbing patterns. I ceased to be for her trustworthy in the way she had got used to. (The therapeutic framework is, I am glad to say, often robust enough to survive these shocks as long as the therapist is capable of being honest about feelings and mistakes, which means being self-accepting.) However, these minutes were stressful for me as well. I had to struggle with what I had done, and with Lesley's anger. I needed to recognize three truths:

- I, Richard, deserved her anger, because I had got it wrong for her.
- I, Richard, did not deserve my own anger, because I cannot be some sort of 'gold-standard' counsellor who never makes a mistake. Counsellor perfectionism leads to neurotic rigidity (Tudor and Worrall, 2004, pp. 5–6).
- I had ceased for a while to be Richard for Lesley and had become another version of her mother.

In a tight corner, I needed something to hang onto that would steady me. On this occasion it was the sense of having stirred up for Lesley a transferential element to our relationship. On the spot, I could albeit vaguely name this to myself. It was like having a road map at a scary point on the journey. However, my scrap of a map is also controversial. While I suspect that some person-centred rejection of others' theories is mere tribalism, there is much intelligent criticism of the bases of other approaches. Ellingham (2005) offers an important critique of transference. However, theories even when very approximate models of reality remain useful tools. I simply note of transference as I use the idea here that it provided me with a framework which helped me remain calm in the face of my own error, and so not move towards the punitive, 'maternal' stance that I might have found. In other words, reference within me to one single theory could have rendered me defensive and hence abusive of the client. As it happened, I was able to remain open to what I had inadvertently done as a reality-for-Lesley to be worked with.

In the coming chapters, other theories will be invoked for a number of reasons. There will be a range of insights available. How these affect the counselling relationship, and how they influence the counsellor's interventions is similarly variable. The key principle is to remain aware of the phenomenological basis of therapy and the actualizing tendency of the client.

## Into Practice

- Careful and respectful listening is founded on the fact that it is impossible to know the client's world, unless we put in painstaking and cautious effort to build up our comprehension, in both head and heart.
- Listen to your own prejudices. Know them. They are not wrong, bad or unprofessional. What you do with them is what matters. Bracket them out: 'I know I think this, but I will wait until I become wiser in my client's world.' Bracketing out can be about understanding the client, or it can be about our according unconditional positive regard. It is respectful to bracket out my judging of the client.
- Give the client's material equal weight. Do this inside yourself. Some practitioners aim to give equal weight to what they reflect verbally; others give a greater emphasis to focusing and responding selectively. I tend to be more attentive to horizontalizing my responses in the earlier days of a relationship, or when the client feels unsafe, or when I feel somehow lost. Inside, avoid judgements about what the client's world is 'really' like.
- The client's world is made up of a number of elements. These include thoughts, feelings, beliefs, cultural and religious contexts, life-decisions, scripts, bodily sensations, ways of looking at relationships, connections made and unmade, the degree of awareness of thoughts and feelings, and much more. They all form the client's world or frame of reference. Listen for these with equal weight, as far as you can. What is important amongst these for your client?
- However, it is impossible to be aware of all of these equally. Empathy includes estimating which of these might be important for your client.
- Your client's frame of reference is many-layered. Different layers change at different paces. Some ways of my looking at my world need five years to alter; at other times my perspective shifts second by second. Be alert to this.
- Be prepared to work at the edge of your client's awareness.
- Therapy involves changes in the way clients put their world together. Some alter consciously, by thinking through, for example, their conditions of

worth; others change largely by adapting out of awareness but within the therapeutic relationship. Be alert to the way your client does this. It will deeply affect what you reflect to them.

- Explore connections. Do not presume that what makes sense to you will make sense to your client. In change, feelings often go before understanding.
- When a client is changing, he will be stressed and sometimes frightened. Be prepared to give support and challenge in response to the client's level of stress or fear. Be wary of trusting your own feelings about where the client is. Listen. Ask.
- That of which neither of you is conscious may be more important than what you think you know about the client.
- Be prepared to allow other counselling theories, particularly those rooted in the phenomenological perspective, to inform you of *how* your client might be thinking, feeling or processing. However, never believe what a theory tells you without checking it out with your client.

I invite you in reading the coming chapters to broaden your understanding of process. In Chapter 13 threads of this understanding will be drawn together in a consideration of the work of Greenberg *et al.* (1993).

## Further Reading

Baker, N. (2007) *The Experiential Counselling Primer*. Ross-on-Wye, PCCS Books.

This book is a clear and impressive introduction to experiential therapy, from a British author who gets less attention for his work than he deserves. This is an important little book, and complements well the current volume. Baker is less radical then Greenberg, for example.

Becker, C.S. (1992) *Living and Relating: An Introduction to Phenomenology*. London, Sage.

Carol Becker combines an introduction to the principles and practice of phenomenologically informed psychology with an account of human development. It is a good alternative to Ernesto Spinelli's account, below. Her illustrations are helpful and link to lifespan development in a way I find useful.

Greenberg, L.S., L.N. Rice and R. Elliott (1993) *Facilitating Emotional Change: The Moment-by-Moment Process*. New York, The Guilford Press.

This is a very demanding text. A summary of it appears in Chapter 13 of this volume. However, it is a masterly account of the relation of phenomenology to the integration of person-centred and Gestalt therapies. It then goes on to illustrate what Jerold Bozarth has called the specificity fallacy: if you can describe what is wrong, you can match this to a specific treatment. I describe above the myth of pseudo-science that the more objective a thing is the more accurately we have grasped it. The second half of this book is a good example of this myth.

Lietaer, G. (1998) 'From Non-Directive to Experiential: A Paradigm Unfolding' in Thorne and Lambers (1998), 62–73.

This is a classical, brief and important statement of the process-orientated approach from within a European perspective. Lietaer raises in a short space some key issues, while having a different approach to them from the current author.

Spinelli, E. (1989/2005) *The Interpreted World: Introduction to Phenomenological Psychology.* London, Sage.

The fullest account of the relationship between psychology, counselling and phenomenology which also remains accessible to students and practising counsellors alike. Spinelli's own practice, which he terms existential, is very close indeed to person-centred practice.

Worsley, R. (2007) *The Integrative Counselling Primer.* Ross-on-Wye, PCCS Books.

A useful way to begin to think about phenomenology as the basis for integration in person-centred practice. This is the basis of the penultimate section of this chapter.

# 5

# Constructing the Self: Narrative and Metaphor in Therapy

In this chapter, I explore the narrating of the self as an aspect of client process. The client's act of narrating is a key aspect of her process. The act is not the same as the content of a narrative. The content may even be inconsequential, although that is unlikely. The act of telling is itself a constituting of identity. In this context, I also describe Mearns and Thorne's (2000) work on configurations of the self, in that psychotherapy generally is now much more prone to think of the self as multiple, and hence of personal identity as a way of managing this multiplicity. The relationship between the different configurations is itself a narrative process.

## A Letter to Alistair

> Internal communication is clear, with feelings and symbols well matched, and fresh terms for new feelings. There is an experience of effective choice of new ways of being.
>
> (Rogers, 1957c, in Rogers, 1967, p. 154)

In Rogers (1957c), one of the key indicators of the fully functioning person is that there is adequate symbolization of feeling and, indeed, I would add, of all significant, internal processing. It is a key element of client process and of psychological change that the client tells her story afresh. This can happen time and again, or it can appear as a single transformative event. This chapter aims to explore a little of the role of narrative in client process.

It is usual for the client to tell her own story and for the therapist to reflect this *ex tempore* in person-centred therapy. From time to time, a more structured approach is useful.

I can imagine that some would protest at the idea that the story might emerge from the therapist as well as the client. Is this being faithful to the client's frame of reference? I draw attention to a passage from Rogers (1970):

> Or the intuition may be a bit more complex. While a responsible business executive is speaking, I may suddenly have the fantasy of the small boy that he was, shy, inadequate, fearful – a child he endeavours to deny, of whom he is ashamed. And I am wishing that he may love and cherish this youngster. So I may voice this fantasy – not as something true but as a fantasy within me.
>
> (Rogers, 1970, p. 53)

In this passage, Rogers relates his use of his own intuitive capacity to be with his client through creating an image within himself, and then sharing it with the client. In the shared creation of the client's story, a similar process is afoot, although on a larger scale. As ever, there must be before the therapist the question: do I understand as fully as I can how it is for you – the patterns, the feelings, the symbols, the meanings?

I wrote the following letter to Alistair with his prior agreement, as a piece of miniature, phenomenological research.

---

**Case 5.1 A letter to Alistair**

Dear Alistair,

It was good to see you again last week. I was struck as we worked together how perhaps for the first time. I was beginning to get a sense of pattern, of large-scale meaning surfacing in what we have been talking about together. I was grateful that you agreed to let me put down on paper what I think I was hearing, so that you could respond to it if you want.

Throughout the number of months in which we have been meeting, I have been mindful of your intermittent feelings of depression. I have also been struck by the fact that your job as a priest in a difficult York-shire mining community – with the separation between church and so many in the community, with the sense of apathy and at times alien-ation of which you have spoken – would leave many a priest feeling discouraged. I also recognize that you have told me about your sense of having to prove your worth within your childhood home. But today, for the first time I think I became aware of a pattern in your life; at least that is how it seemed to me.

Perhaps it was made clearer by the contrast between the depressed feelings that went with your recent bout of flu and your buoyant feelings – or perhaps more grittily determined and purposeful than buoyant – which you had when we met a few days ago. I guess that you have seen how not being able to work can leave you aimless and feeling confused and perhaps even in touch with a sense of worthlessness. I felt that it would have been easy for me to see your renewed energy as just a revitalized defence against depression. However, that felt to be far too simplistic. I sensed in you last week a vein of joy at your own vigour.

I was particularly struck by your speaking of living your life backwards. While most people aim to move forward towards success, you felt that you had moved towards an outer set of circumstances in which success was more and more denied to you, at least in obvious terms. We both know how other clergy have appreciated your ability to look realistically at the sense of failure that can come with pastoral ministry.

Your story of your adult life seems to me to have fallen for you into three parts so far – and that begs the question as to where it is going now – a new stage?

During the first stage, you were a lay missionary. You experienced your work as 'going with the flow' of the culture of Africa. You lived in a harsh and isolated environment, with no chance of getting away from the work setting, and with very real pressures for Pam with young children. However, your teaching and your pastoral work were welcomed and affirmed very strongly. It's not like that in England today! It struck me that the combination of isolation and success felt quite an incentive to engage with work at every possible time, and not to switch off.

Coming back to England meant theological training and then a curacy. Amidst all that you have told me, I have been struck by the fact that your real skills abroad were simply not valued by others – or at least that is how it has felt to you. You were a theological teacher who was then taught by others, and sometimes this felt a bad experience. You became a curate and had difficult colleague relationships. You felt frustrated by this, and again undervalued. Above all, you pushed yourself hard to keep coping.

In the years you have been in your present parish, you have felt a considerable change in yourself, although it has been covered over by times of depression. I was particularly struck by your renewed appreciation of your now grown-up children and your pleasure in them, as well as a new determination to enjoy the present moment with Pam. No longer are you waiting for retirement before relaxation can be claimed. You have been struggling to get a new perspective through your doctoral research into the sociology of the church's marginalization in your parish. It feels like it is no longer good enough to blame yourself. The church can be a source of despair but also of hope – a new sense of being focused.

When the time is ripe for you to move on, you now feel that you can go without worrying about being seen as a failure there. In a difficult environment, it seems as if you have been, as you might say, experimenting with failure in order to take the sting out of it, to detoxify it.

And so, a new stage emerging? I wonder if you could let me know if I have got anywhere near your own perceptions of your personal story.

Richard.

## *Reflection*

> The reason for meeting the client at relational depth is that at that intensity of relating the client may give us invited access into his existential Self. He is giving us access to the innermost feelings and thoughts about his Self and his very existence. He is not giving us a false picture layered with conscious defences and pretences – he is including the therapist in the inner dialogue he has with himself. More than that, he is including the therapist in the moment-to-moment discoveries he is making about his Self while he is at the very 'edge of awareness'.
>
> (Mearns, 1999, p. 125)

Over many months of work with me, Alistair has engaged with his own lack of self-worth. He has been able to identify this intellectually and retrieve memories and feelings from his childhood, re-experiencing something of the pressures from a home background that was loving but severe. He described his childhood as characterized by a deep faith in God – and a commitment to joylessness. He has felt what my letter described as ' a joy at your own vigour'. I now would rephrase this as 'the vigour of his own joy'. Alistair's conditions of worth were bound up not only with his need to achieve, to conform, but the requirement that he should do all of this joylessly.

He has never conformed to this last requirement. He has always sought out some form of rebellious joy. He told of times when his affections were rebutted by Pam. At no point was he discouraged, but persisted until he changed her mind about him. Alistair has been able to develop an aspect of his self-concept that, at worst, might seem to others arrogant. He never conceived of her not liking him in the end; in a sense there was nothing to lose. It was not a hollow arrogance, but a joyful questing in hope. ('Why am I not more like that?' he would ask.) Rogers has spoken of our actualizing aspects of the self-concept which are in fact conditioned but functional. There is a gap between the functional and the fully functioning. I suggest that Alistair's quest for joy not only represents an organismic aspect of himself, but is also the actualizing of this conditioned aspect of himself. He seeks joy because it was unacceptably forbidden. However, he always has done so in the setting of his need to please himself and others by conforming and succeeding. The healthy urge for joy is set in the context of his wider conditions of worth, and so, while very good in itself, is contaminated by the surrounding elements of his self-concept. The result is a stubbornness which can, from my perspective, vary from the admirably tenacious and courageous to the irritating.

This description of Alistair, I hope, gives a flavour of the role in self-actualization that depression has. The person-centred therapist needs to be clear about her view of depression. Severe (often called, quite unhelpfully, clinical) depression is disabling, at times even becoming psychotic. In spite of this, I want to suggest that depression is in some of its manifestations life-promoting in the long run. It is essentially evidence that we are taking seriously in our whole selves the tensions between our need to self-actualize and the restrictions felt from our past life-scripts.

Alistair's depression is a defence against the paranoid feelings of repression by the Calvinistic element of his upbringing. It is a symbolizing of the frustration of his desire to actualize his need for guilt-free joy through deeply *self*-evaluating processes, rather than through parental and hence external evaluation.

Thus, we return to the story, the narrative. Alistair's response to my letter was cursory. It felt to me as if a brief reading did not produce a Damascus-road enlightenment, but a simple and familiar recognition and hence a desire to move on – a carrying forward of the story and its attached images into Alistair's own self-understanding, at the levels of both thinking and feeling. As I write, I know that at some appropriate point I want to check this out further with Alistair.

Supposing that it was of use, then one function of Alistair's telling his story has been in our recognizing together the underlying pattern: I have lived my life backwards. Alistair first learned to seek the joy he needed. Then he has systematically moved into more and more testing situations, with the result that the joy was no longer a defence against low self-esteem but now exists even where tough reality assails self-worth.

No doubt I have a skewed rendering of his story in my mind, but the upshot in general is that Alistair has, quite unconsciously, structured his life to confront his demons. His actualizing tendency has enabled him to face not only his need for joy in the face of parental disapproval, but also his deeper and more testing need to experience difficulty, even persecution, without losing a grasp of either joy or reality. Depression is a stage in the story; the narrative symbolizes its working-through. The seeing of dysfunction as positive is inherent in the concept of the actualizing tendency. However, it has been emphasized in recent years by increased mutual understanding between psychotherapy and the positive psychology movement.

In recent years, there has been a growing appreciation of the synergy between the person-centred approach and the discipline of positive psychology (Linley and Joseph, 2004; Joseph and Worsley, 2005; Joseph and Linley, 2006; Worsley and Joseph, 2007; Levitt, 2008). This rapprochement has been led in the United Kingdom to a great extent by Stephen Joseph, who combines being a Professor of Psychology, Health and Social Care at the University of Nottingham with being a client-centred therapist. Stephen Joseph, together with his co-workers, has introduced positive psychology to the counselling world, but with a particular twist to it.

In the United States, Martin Seligman had, since 1999, alerted psychologists to the need to understand the positive in human experience as well as the clinically dysfunctional (Joseph and Linley, 2006, pp. 1–4). In other words, psychologists had spent too much energy on examining what goes wrong with human mental experience, and so had failed to grasp what the strengths are. The obvious application of this might be to find ways to motivate people in the work place. Joseph, with others, has consistently linked this focus on positive experience with the core theory of Carl Rogers, and in particular the actualizing tendency. It is characteristic of Joseph's emphasis on positive psychology *in practice*, psychology as positive therapy, that we are invited to call into question the notion that all that a client experiences as distress is, in the long run, negative. We actualize our potential as best we might, at times in very adverse circumstances. Sometimes what is actualized falls a long way short of the ideal – whatever that might be. However, what is actualized includes a positive focus. This is all too easy for therapists to miss, because they are dysfunction-attuned, to back away from for fear of being insensitive in suggesting that painful experience may have an up side. When we miss the positive, we inadvertently deprive our clients of a possible resource. Thus, in the case of Alistair, it became to be of great encouragement to him that he had confronted the demons of his own upbringing, on the way through life, even if that had not generated a so-called complete 'cure'.

The importance of the hidden positive in clients' experience is even more telling in the case of Emma. I set out a brief summary, below, but a far fuller account can be read in Worsley and Joseph (2007, chapter 9.)

---

**Case 5.2   Emma**

Emma, a young academic, who taught English literature, came to see me because she had suffered from chronic depression for many years, and had been hospitalized in her late teens. She was remarkably stuck in her depression. We worked together for some three years – about a hundred sessions. Something felt very 'locked in'. She was chronically unable to confront her image of herself as possibly healthy. Guilt kept this at bay. Had she believed that she might be content, at ease and guilt-free, she would have needed to acknowledge the role of her family over four generations in her deep distress. Work with Emma felt like circling again and again through the same despair, with little obvious sign of progress. As part of this, I began to challenge Emma to consider that she might be a deeply functional person even if she continued to feel depressed from time to time. Her distress need not define her. I was uncertain whether this connected with anything within her.

One of Emma's characteristic fears was of hell-fire, even though she no longer practised the faith of her teenage years. This symbolized her self-hatred, and so was not at all open to rational encounter. It too was stuck fast. Emma taught medieval and renaissance literature, by and large. The fear of hell-fire made Dante's *Divine Comedy* and Milton's *Paradise Lost*, for instance, very painful texts to encounter.

One day, I commented rather quizzically – maybe out of my own frustration with Emma's stuckness – that I was surprised that she has opted for medieval rather than modern literature, where the theme of hell appears less frequently. She looked at me firmly, and commented that it was better to be alive with Milton and Dante than deadened by the hand of Samuel Beckett. In other words, some years previously, Emma had already made the existential decision to live even if she suffered than to enter into an intellectually and spiritually vacuous state, as she saw it.

## Narrative as Symbolization

Rogers (1957c) stresses the importance of symbolizing internal experience in those who are becoming more fully functioning. Why? His observation is a pragmatic one. That is what he saw happening. However, the person who symbolizes accurately becomes more deeply congruent. When I look symbolically at how I am, I can own and experience myself less defendedly.

A surface example of this springs to mind. It was one of my joys as a teacher of counselling to attempt to teach Freud in a handful of hours to a class of nurses-to-be. The Oedipus complex is fun. Of course, we chaps have never had sexual desires for our mothers, have we? Sigmund is a bit of a weirdo! It's all a bit sick. So I tell them Frank O'Connor's (1963) wonderful story – 'My Oedipus Complex'. It is an enchanting tale of a little boy whose father returns from war. In such recognizable terms we see and feel his immense jealousy.

How could his mother be such a fool as to fall for this man? One day, he will grow up and marry his mother and they will have children. Then another child arrives – 17s 6d from the hospital. Father is now also cast out by the screaming newcomer. He appears in son's bed, furious. Son asks for a cuddle. Father seems awkward for some reason, but complies. The boy reflects, 'He is rather bony, but better than nothing.'

When Freud's theory is adequately symbolized as narrative, our defences are overcome and we recognize a portrayal of aspects of our own experience. In respect of our infant sexuality, we become more congruent.

Story is an extended metaphor. It draws comparisons between our internal processes and our thinking and language. Metaphor and story keep us sane. Ben Knights (1995) puts it like this:

> Those who listen to and counsel others are again and again in the presence of matters quite literally of life and death. For the personality to sustain this and to go on being of use ... requires ... considerable inner resources. It is my intuition that such resources cannot be imagined just as serene inner space, but rather that one must see inner space itself as a stage on which the transformative power of symbols is experienced.
>
> (Knights, 1995, p. 2)

What is true for the therapist is even more so for the client. Story and metaphor can people the stage of our inner life with richness which includes keys to life's meaning for us.

Our current understanding of metaphor is deeply influenced by the work of the modern French philosopher, Paul Ricoeur, and in particular his book, *The Rule of Metaphor* (Brown, 1987; Clark, 1990). For Ricoeur, metaphor is neither an addition nor an embellishment to literal meaning, and certainly not a rhetorical decoration. As his commentator S.H. Clark says, 'There are no metaphorical words, only metaphorical utterances, and no deviations from a literal meaning, only an operation of predication' (Clark, 1990, p. 123).

In other words, metaphor is not a 'thing' but a way of acting with language. Metaphor is a radical linking of two elements of literal language. It is this linking or predication which is the heart of metaphor. In metaphor, says Ricoeur, there is always a surplus of meaning. The meaning of a metaphor goes way beyond what can ever be retrieved by a single reading. It incorporates the conscious intention of speaker and hearer, some of their unconscious material and parts of the life-force of the culture in which speaker and hearer co-exist. Ricoeur's point is that this is not a happy accident; the richness of metaphor is about the deep nature of reality (Brown, 1987, p. 181). As Husserl had pointed out, the transcendental object, the Thing-in-Itself in the outside world, is finally inexpressible, but not wholly unknowable. Therefore, metaphor expresses in itself some of the hidden qualities of the real object. In other words, metaphor puts out into the world a richness of meaning which goes beyond the conscious knowledge of either speaker or hearer, but which is always there to be discovered by either or both.

Narrative, life-story, is in many ways simply extended metaphor. However, unlike metaphor, narrative has to be told. It is in this *act* of telling that the self reconstitutes itself. In person-centred terms, this would be an important element in the revision of the self-concept and in a consequent increase in congruence. In Alistair's terms, it is when he sees that he has lived his life backwards that he can glimpse the connection between his depressive self and his self-valuing. It is no co-incidence that the re-storying of his life (in part out of awareness) is based upon a key metaphor – 'I have lived my life backwards.'

Clients become more congruent when they locate the therapeutically signif-icant metaphors and narratives by which to live (McLeod, 1997). Language manages both meaning and relationships.

I am grateful to Hobson (1985) for introducing me to part of Rilke's *Duino Elegies* thus:

> [We look for] a language of word-kernels, a language that's not gathered, up above, on stalks, but grasped in the speech-seed ... isn't the pure silence of love like heart-soil around such speech seeds? Oh how often one longs to speak a few degrees more deeply ... a shade further in the ground ... but one gets only a minimal layer further down; one's left with a mere intimation of the kind of speech that may be possible there, where silence reigns.
>
> (Rilke, 1952, translated by J.B. Leishman and
> S. Spender, cited by R. Hobson, 1985, p. 61)

This passage both states and illustrates the depth of language which underlies the rational but exceeds its meanings, feelings, experiencings by far. As we lis-ten, we struggle together with our clients to regain the richness of the language in which more of their truth is spoken than either they or we can at first know.

## Into Practice – 1

There is a question of method in therapy: whose metaphor, whose narrative?

The safe, person-centred answer is the client's. This is naïve and unrealistic. Some therapists work on the basis that the only task is to track the client – half a pace behind. Of course there is evidence that Rogers did not work quite like this, not least the quotation from Rogers (1970) near the beginning of this chapter.

I suggest that metaphor and narrative are radically interpersonal. I will explain what I mean by this below. They share one quality – their meaning is never exhausted – but differ in one key way – narrative belongs to the teller in a way that metaphor does not. This influences how we address narrative and metaphor in therapy.

Let us start with the quality of both: that meaning is never exhausted. Metaphor and narrative can continually invite further consideration, a seeking for more, greater or different meaning. Empathy therefore requires that the therapist is as engaged and puzzled as the client. For much of the time, it is crucial that clients have the room to explore their own meanings and options. It would be a travesty of the phenomenological approach for the therapist to be butting in, interpreting, speculating. Yet there must also be an element of shared play between two people. Metaphor and narrative both have something of the quality of my saying: this is what I mean, and I wonder what that means. They are interpersonal because they invite shared exploration. Often the therapist will facilitate the client's associations and ponderings, but from time to time, as with Rogers, cited above, it will become clear that a congruent response from the therapist, from her own imaginative resourcefulness, will clarify something for the client. It is only another, but very rich, form of asking: is this what you mean? Whether it is a rich resource or an intrusion is not a matter of designing an appropriate intervention. That would be too 'local'. It depends upon the quality of the whole therapeutic relationship. Has the therapist established a power balance that the client can trust as non-intrusive? If so, then she has also given herself room to share her own imaginative responses non-abusively with the client.

The interpersonal quality of metaphor and narrative is not an option. The language by which we live and manage our relating is always between ourselves and others. The therapist offers, as part of her unconditional positive regard for the client, the experience of wrestling with metaphor and story. Without the possibility of that risk the client will not have learned to negotiate meaning with significant others.

The difference between a metaphor and a life-narrative is that the metaphor is one of an infinite number of tropes, while the life-narrative feels like a version of a single and unique story. It belongs more closely to the client. More patient, careful listening is needed; more accurate checking out; less playful exploration; greater care in suggesting 'structures' like 'life lived backwards'. The therapist needs to be more guarded about what she offers from within herself towards the client's life-narrative. One cannot say, as of a metaphor: let's throw it away and start again.

This brief consideration of narrative and metaphor illustrates a truth of person-centred work conducted in awareness of the fact that the client is in process. 'Process' is itself a metaphor for the many and complex events within the client's mind and body which parallel thinking and feeling. As both client and therapist become more congruently familiar with these, then engagement at existential depth becomes possible, for processing involves self-expression in many ways. One process-orientated self-expression is through the engagement of meaning in narrative and metaphor.

Listen, play, respect, be puzzled, together.

# The Multiple Self

However, is there but one story? It has been presumed throughout early modernity that the self is a unity. This was certainly the mindset of Carl Rogers. I want to return to a quotation from Rogers (1970) which I cited above. Rogers imagines that there is a little boy present, who needs nurture. Yet, he consigns this to fantasy within him and *not as something true*. He is right that he cannot inflict it on the client as a truth by way of an abusively powerful interpretation, of course. However, there may be more objective truth to Rogers' fantasy that he was willing to countenance. In recent years, person-centred theory has developed the concept of the self as a complex system in which there are multiples selves in action and reaction. Mearns and Thorne (2000) have termed these configurations of the self, whereas John Rowan (1990) termed them sub-personalities. This work on the plurality of the self has been expanded upon by Mick Cooper (1999), for instance. To return to Rogers' intuition, this move makes the little boy not just a fantasy of Rogers' but also an aspect of the client, a configuration of his self or being. Rogers was not merely entertaining a fantasy about the client, but was (possibly? probably?) in touch with an aspect of the client.

What, then, is a configuration of the self? The following is Mearns' and Thorne's (2000, p. 102) initial, working definition:

> A 'configuration' is a hypothetical construct denoting a coherent pattern of feelings, thoughts and preferred behavioural responses symbolised or pre-symbolised by the person as a reflective dimension of existence within the Self.

I find that I can read this definition at two levels – the first a simple notion of what a configuration is, and the second a more thought-provoking analysis of Mearns and Thorne's carefully chosen words. First, the simple version comes to the fore.

As we talk with clients, we can come to see that underneath confusion and ambivalence can lurk a sense for the client that they hear more than one voice speaking to them from within. More then one client, on identifying this phenomenon of their own internal world, has asked me: Am I mad? It is part of our culture that we are a unity. To learn, to come to feel, that we are not a unity is disturbing. There can be a confusion with dissociative phenomena, often called multiple personality in common parlance, and then further confusion with the 'splitting off' element in the word schizophrenia. I always assure the client that this is not a sign of madness, but is normal. It is merely that we have not understood this normality before. John Rowan (1990) has helped us correct this misapprehension. He reports that during workshops he has run, people are likely to be able to identify on average six configurations, and occasionally as many as 50.

A configuration behaves much like a single, unitary self, in that it thinks, feels and behaves in characteristics ways that other configurations do not necessarily share. The briefest and clearest way into thinking like this is to be found in Mearns (1994a, pp. 12–14). It is the case study of Elizabeth – the Nun and the Little Girl. Parts A and B are these two configurations; Part C is the new configuration that arises in therapy as a way of mediating between the two.

---

### Box 5.1   The Nun and the Little Girl

#### A – The Nun

- I am a caring person and love my clients.
- I don't do enough as a person.
- I love my husband dearly.
- I cry for the pain of the world.
- I don't know why you bother with me.
- I always let people down.
- I do *try* to do the right thing.
- I am just not good enough.
- If only I could get rid of that bad little girl inside me.

#### B – The Little Girl

- I don't really care. I despise my clients.
- I despise myself.
- I despise my husband.
- I am a sham.
- I am going to leave them all (her family).
- I am so, so scared.
- Help me to get out.
- Don't desert me.
- Help me to destroy that pompous nun.

#### C – After Therapy

- I am really struggling with all of this.
- I am getting so tired … so very tired.
- I don't know whether I am going to make it.
- Sometimes I look at myself and it is like a boxing match going on inside me.
- This depression feels totally different from before. It feels much blacker and I feel fully in it rather than fighting it.

---

The Nun and the Little Girl behave as two separate systems of self. Each has a story, a metaphor-set, of its own. To change the noun 'Self' into a verb, each configuration *selfs* in a different way. The C-Part is another configuration which contacts reality in a different way. In line with Rogers'

(1957c), the C-Part is the result of a fuller communication between, and hence symbolization of the content of, the other two configurations.

The theory of configurations of self posits that the self is not unitary, but that each configuration can be bound into its own internal communication-and-process-world at the expense of communicating with both the environment and other configurations. This is a version of the incongruence that Rogers (1957a) describes. However, the concept of configurations has a number of implications for practice. Personal Focus 5.1 is not an exhaustive list of these, but rather a suggestive list. We each need to think this through for ourselves within our practice.

---

**Personal Focus 5.1　Configurations in Practice**

*What follows is a number of thoughts to consider, and not rules that ought to be followed. The list is far from exhaustive:*

1. Be aware that some clients associate multiple notions of the self with some sort of oddity or madness. Does the client know that multiple configurations are normal?
2. Do not impose the idea of a particular configuration. Negotiate it. Is it from the client's frame of reference or yours? How does this matter?
3. Accord the core conditions to all configurations. This is called multidirectional partiality (Mearns and Cooper, 2005, pp. 122–4).
4. Are you aware of how the different configurations communicate, one with another? What might be the blocks?
5. Are some of the configurations orientated against the client's growth?
6. Can you facilitate dialogue between configurations? How?
7. Take care that the client is safe enough in the work that you are doing. Check this out from time to time. Does it feel OK? Does it make sense to them? Is it too scary?
8. Does it make sense to think of different configurations having their own narratives or life-stories?
9. How do the client's configurations fit with your own? This is the most testing of these thoughts in practice. See Mearns and Thorne (2000, pp. 138–140) for a useful exercise in being aware of one's own pattern of configurations.

---

All of this is based on a first, simple reading of Mearns' and Thorne's definition, above. A closer reading bears fruit.

# Configurations Revisited – Narrative and Metaphor

Mearns and Thorne's (2000) definition is not only an initial, working definition. It is both carefully considered and rather cautious. I want to focus upon
one part of it only:

> ...a hypothetical construct denoting a coherent pattern of feelings,
> thoughts and preferred behavioural responses...

This is both a cautious and difficult phrase. I understand easily enough the
notion of a coherent pattern of thoughts, feelings and responses. It is the first
four words that trouble me. A hypothetical construct is a structured idea which
is held by someone as a way of thinking, as a first guess at something. A hypothesis is the statement of alleged fact that is to be tested in an experiment, for
instance. The words 'hypothetical construct' locate the configuration firmly
within the mind of Mearns and Thorne, or the therapist, or even of the client
thinking about herself. Another hypothetical construct might begin: Let us
suppose for a minute that I am a cat. I am not a cat. Another might begin: Let
us suppose for a minute that I am an economist. It is reasonable to think that I
am the latter but not the former, except for some strange thought experiment.
What precisely is denoted? (Denotation is often seen as a literal statement
which points to the real.)

There are, I think, two possible answers to this question. I happen to believe
that both are true, and in working with configurations I find it helpful to
remember both.

*A configuration is a metaphor.* In an obvious sense, I take this to be the
case. Elizabeth never was actually a nun. 'The Nun' is a name given to an
aspect of her that has allegedly nun-like qualities. (We could argue that real
nuns were rarely like this, but the metaphor still works.) It is an extended act
of reference. If this is the case, then all the things that have been said above
about narratives and metaphors apply to configurations too. In a broad sense, I
can ask a client: Do you feel this metaphor fits? It continues to be the case that
the client is the expert in the answer to this question. The idea of fit is akin to
the idea of felt-sense or felt-meaning. The client who was asked this question
tries to match the metaphor to perhaps a conscious idea but almost certainly
to an incompletely symbolized but physically experienced (in the guts, as we
say!) 'feel' of what makes sense (Gendlin, 1996, 1997). The configuration is a
hypothesis – educated guess – about an image or story that functions to make
sense in the client's life. It is useful in precisely the same way that all metaphors
and narratives are useful.

However, I want to move beyond and ask, but where does the configuration exist? If it is a hypothetical construct, then it exists in the discourse
between therapist and client. It is something we talk about. It is as useful as
the talk itself. Yet, in the next section I want to think about working with

configurations that *are not* talked about. This can only make sense if the configuration refers to something that exists as an object-in-the-world, and not as a metaphor. This would mean that a configuration is more than an idea. It is a reality in the client's brain. I mean this in a quite specific way. Of course even the metaphor of the nun is encoded in the client's neural activity *as metaphor*. The code is physical, but the metaphor is of course not. I want to propose that the configuration can be thought of as physical, as neural too. This means that there is a subsystem of the brain which corresponds in some way to 'The Nun'.

At this point life gets complex. We are in the area of neuroscience and the biology of mind. We must be wary of being too slick here. It takes great academic courage to reach the conclusion that we have very little idea about the nature of human consciousness (Gray, 2004). We can fool ourselves that we know more than we do. Neuroscience is a popular theme in counselling at the moment. It needs to be taken on board cautiously. It seems to me that all too often references to neuroscience are used as a drunk uses a lamp post – more for support than illumination. They function to give pseudo-scientific credibility to parts of the psychological pursuit. With this warning in place, I want to offer one particular model of brain activity which is rooted in Darwinian neurobiology, and which I find useful. It comes from Gerald Edelman's (1992) book, *Bright Air, Brilliant Fire*.

Edelman is a neuroscientist who won the Nobel Prize in 1972. Like Gray (2004), he stresses our need to be humble about what we know. However, he offers a way of thinking about consciousness that is useful. His basic idea about higher consciousness – the reflexive awareness we have of past and future, history and meaning – is that it involves a highly complex and multi-layered process which he terms *high-level, global re-entrant mapping* (Edelman, 1992, p. 89). He posits the idea that the emergence of self depends upon a process in which the brain constructs identity through a continuous mapping or cataloguing of its own lower-level cortical functions. He calls it re-entrant mapping because it is as if the higher-level systems has the ability to tap back into lower-level systems and then construct maps of them and other related systems.

If Edelman is anywhere near the truth at all, he is describing a complex process which would make the notion of configurations more than hypothetical constructs. It is possible that a configuration is closely related to a system of mapping within the brain. Why is this important?

If we look back to the diagram of the Nun and the Little Girl, above, we can see that there emerges through therapy a new configuration – the C-Part. The Nun and the Little Girl continue to be – at least for a while. We may want to think of them as books in a library which become consulted less and less frequently as they get out-of-date. In Edelman's terms, the C-Part is one version of self which mediates between other parts. In other words, the increased congruence presumes that there comes to be a new level of communication between different configurations. This communication looks like a change to the mapping process. It is the removal of denial of experience and of the remembered past.

A metaphor cannot do this. In any case many clients change inwardly like Elizabeth without the process of change becoming 'directly' conscious. There are likely to be complex brain–mind structures which change, which learn to communicate more widely. Edelman's model helps us to see how this might be. This is important as we come to think about configurations which exist but are not constructs as they are not referred to in the therapy.

## Into Practice – 2

At one level, thinking about configurations of self looks like getting into a particular language pattern or game. We need, we might think, to talk about named aspects of the client. In their case study of Jim, for example, Mearns and Thorne (2000, pp. 101–8) describe three configurations marked as 'Guardian', 'Bastard' and 'sad and lonely part'. It is tempting particularly for the less experienced counsellor to want to get into this talk. It can feel powerful, like delivering the goods or using a new technique. This would be contrary to the heart and soul of person-centred practice. Work with configurations of self need not even involve this labelling. It is first of all an awareness within the therapist that there is more than one set of feelings, more than one grammar, more than one narrative or metaphor at play within the client. These configurations show characteristic patterns of communication and non-communication within and between themselves. However, the therapist cannot presume that she knows or can plot these accurately. Premature naming of them can set in stone something which is either not right or merely passing.

I therefore want to give an example of a moment of therapy which is simple on the surface, and in which 'thinking' configurations precedes their naming.

---

**Case 5.3  Angélique**

Angélique worked as an assistant bank manager and came to see me in private practice. Although she was professionally competent, as far as I could tell, she was constantly anxious and from time to time paranoid. She had recently bought a nearly new car, well within her financial circumstances. However, she was obsessed with concerns about it breaking down, being a death trap or otherwise betraying her. She recognized that this was not reasonable, but rather was out of proportion. In our initial interview, I had gained the impression that she was the younger daughter of a caring but anxious and self-deprecating mother.

As the first two sessions progressed, I quickly realized that I should not use the word paranoid too lightly of Angélique. A number of increasingly exotic stories emerged about her workplace. It felt to her as if many others in the office were against her, and, with the best will in the world, I found it very difficult to believe all that she said to me. Between the second and the third sessions I checked out with my supervisor what grounds, if any, I had to get Angélique to be seen by our local Early Intervention in Psychosis Team. We agreed that this was not yet appropriate.

First, Angélique functioned well enough at work despite her bizarre perceptions of others. Secondly, it became clear to me that Angélique still had a fairly clear access to her own process on many occasions. There was indeed a part of Angélique which was paranoid, and which distorted her perceptions of others. I could estimate that her mother had left her with something of a dilemma in life. Mother was both overwhelmingly anxious and very scared of being seen to achieve. This was not feminine – but I guessed it was what she had wanted in the past. Therefore, Angélique lived with the double bind of her father's expectation that she should do well after taking a Business Studies degree and her mother's terror of 'being successful', which on the surface meant unfeminine, but underneath meant being saddled with responsibilities that were unbearable.

One configuration exhibited the full disturbance that this engendered double bind – her paranoid self. However, there were other aspects of her which were not only more rooted in reality and emotional maturity, but which could recognize the paranoia for what it was. It would sometimes take her a number of days to recognize that her thinking was paranoid. (I notice the difference between her and me is that I can do this in hours, not days.) In the room, I could experience sometimes being in touch with the paranoid part of her, and at other times with a far more contactful aspect. Both seemed remarkably plausible at the time.

When I thought of her as in paranoid presentation – and of course I could never be certain on any given occasion – I chose not to challenge her thinking, but to remain with what I took to be the underlying fear and distress. However, when I was in touch with the other part of her, I maintained a firm sense of what I thought and what she thought to be real and what the result of her paranoia. In this mode, she could check her own reality.

The outcome, in brief, was that Angélique became more functional at work, although the improvement was not too astounding. However, she learned to relate to the aspect of herself that had paranoid thoughts, and to see it as the logical outcome of her mother's anxiety. Always it was the case that neither Angélique nor I were totally certain of where the paranoia began and ended.

## Reflection

What is unusual about Angélique is that she had remained high-functioning by confining the madness to one aspect of herself. I had come across this in a number of clients in the past. In particular, I was aware of the writing of Kay Redfield Jamison (1993), in which she offers an eloquent account not only of the creative aspect of bipolar disorder, but especially of her own ability to use colleagues to check out her level of functioning from time to time.

Had I been too clumsy in naming the configurations, I might have even damaged the ability of the paranoid one to contain the madness and of the remaining ones to relate to both the paranoia and to her past. Yet, the configuration presented had a major effect on what I thought I needed to do in response. The paranoid part required understanding at the level of feeling, with the hope that it would be able to forge a link eventually between what it felt and Angélique's relationship with her mother. The other aspect of her drew from me a more cognitive and challenging approach, to facilitate her recognizing her paranoia more accurately and living with it creatively. Again, the insights of positive psychology remind us that the structure of seemingly very dysfunctional people can be a brave accommodation of severe distress to creative living. Angélique needed, above all, that her paranoid self, and indeed her whole self, should be respected as a successful woman. Pathologization would have been destructive.

While this case study of Angélique is about configurations of the self, in this chapter, it links closely to the contents of Chapter 12 of this book, in which I consider how the work of Garry Prouty and of Margaret Warner with people with psychosis can also inform our work with normal range client-groups.

Paying close and respectful attention to the narrative and metaphors which comprise the multiple configurations of the client is at the heart of a classically person-centred striving to understand the client's frame of reference. The contents of the next two chapters look towards the possibility of integrating into the therapist's awareness insights from the phenomenological theory of Transactional Analysis and Gestalt therapy.

# Further Reading

## Narrative

Etherington, K. (2000) *Narrative Approaches to Working with Adult Male Survivors of Child Sexual Abuse: The Clients', the Counsellor's and the Researcher's Story.* London, Jessica Kingsley.

Professor Etherington is one of Britain's prime researchers in narrative and therapy. Her book sets out how she works in practice with her theories of narrative. This is an important book. I would however urge the reader not to see 'narrative therapy' as being a model of therapy. The point is that narrative is important in all modalities.

McLeod, J. (1997) *Narrative and Psychotherapy.* London, Sage.

A comprehensive guide to narrative approaches in different therapy approaches. Particular attention can be paid to chapter six, in which the practical means and consequences of the use of narrative to retrieve meaning is spelled out.

McNamee, S. and K.J. Gergen (eds.) (1992) *Therapy as Social Construction.* London, Sage.

We construct our selves from the stories we tell about ourselves. These essays explain the theory behind this process of social construction. It is of practical use in therapy as well as of theoretical interest.

## Configurations of self

The best and simplest introduction to this area of theory remains:

Cooper, M. (1999) 'If you can't be Jekyll be Hyde: an existential-phenomenological exploration of lived-plurality'. In J. Rowan and M. Cooper (eds.) *The Plural Self.* London, Sage, pp. 51–70.
Mearns, D. (1994a) *Developing Person-Centred Counselling.* London, Sage, pp. 12–16.

This brief case study of Elizabeth, while now quite out of date in some ways, is also a very direct illustration of working with configurations of self.

Mearns, D. and B. Thorne (2000) *Person-Centred Therapy Today: New Frontiers in Theory and Practice.* London, Sage, chapters 6 and 7.

# 6

# Conditions of Worth in Everyday Life: A Person-Centred Use of Transactional Analysis Theory

Person-Centred process work is one aspect of empathy. In seeking to understand how a client processes, I am exploring with her one dimension of her world and her activity within it. Often processing is outside of focused awareness. From time to time, awareness will move its light-beam onto processing. This can happen either because the client becomes aware of this part of her experience spontaneously, or because the therapist directs her attention towards this experiencing. In practice, accurate therapy is likely to be a combination or balancing of these.

In this chapter and the next, I explore the possibility of integrating other phenomenological theory with person-centred practice, whilst maintaining the primary and the secondary principles of the Chicago position statement (Sanders, 2000).

The case study of Christopher will be the platform from which to examine the use of ego-state theory from Transactional Analysis (T.A.). I offer this as a useful way of seeing conditions of worth as lived out interpersonally. Classical person-centred theory does not deal so eloquently with the interpersonal aspects of this. The case study illustrates how this sort of conceptualization can promote a process of internal supervision within the therapist. Without ego-state theory I would have understood my reactions to Christopher less well. In gaining a better understanding I was able to challenge his processing of his internalized conditions creatively. At the end of the chapter I offer guidelines for practice. These address the question which is fundamental to the integration of other theory into a full-blooded, person-centred approach: Can I use this understanding in a person-centred way?

The challenge to the reader is to risk venturing outside the beaten track of known and familiar theory. Knowing only person-centred theory does not make you person-centred. One senior colleague read this chapter and complained that I could have done it 'without the T.A.'. The pressure of orthodoxy can make us simply miss the point. To be person-centred is to leave the ghetto.

Let us begin with Christopher.

---

**Case 6.1   Christopher**

> The expense of spirit in a waste of shame
> Is lust in action....
> Enjoyed no sooner but despiséd straight;
> Past reason hunted, and no sooner had,
> Past reason hated, as a swallowed bait
> On purpose laid to make the taker mad.
>
> (Shakespeare, Sonnet 129)

Christopher was a priest in his mid-forties – just a few years younger than me. He was of a Catholic persuasion within the Church of England, a tradition in which priests are sometimes called to a life of celibacy. He had never married, although once he had been engaged.

He presented with depression, and very anxious that I should keep his visits to me confidential from his bishop. He gradually began to relate a string of brief trysts with younger women. On some occasions there was a genuine friendship. He would always end these relationships himself, often after a period of intense sexual activity, in which he became disgusted and appalled at the force of what he persistently called his own lust. On other occasions, there were one-night stands, impersonal and anonymous. He took great care never to get involved with a parishioner. His sexual encounters were kept well clear of his formal work. However, these rash and desperate encounters were also marked by his refusal to practise safer sex, in spite of his fear of disease. I sensed his pleasure in fear, and his fear of pleasure, mingled with a self-destructive force from within him.

I was struck from the early part of our work together by my own torrent of emotion. I wanted to protect him from my disapproval, but also from my acceptance. Above all I felt a flood of almost maternal compassion for his powerlessness.

Christopher had been brought up on a council estate in Wolverhampton. Both of his parents were Irish Protestants. His mother was seemingly warm but his father was puritanical and brutal. He had a sister eight years older and a brother three years younger. His sister had got pregnant when she was 19. She was seen as a disgrace by her father, who disowned her, and to whom she has still found no road back. Her parents parted temporarily at this point. When mother and her two sons returned to be reconciled, father became even more violent and strict. Christopher was struck by his moralized crudeness: 'There'll be no more shagging around in this house, boy.' Christopher found himself, looking back, seeking attention from this man by a combination of playful humour and strict obedience. Neither really worked. In his late teens, this quiet boy had found in his local parish church an acceptance and ethos very different from his father's harsh piety. He began to develop a friendship with a young house-painter in his twenties. Father had berated him lest he be 'queer' – and thus even worse than his sister.

Christopher recalls no feelings or desires or behaviour commensurate with his being gay or bisexual – saving one bout of mutual masturbation with a friend at the age of ten. Yet in retrospect, he sees his engagement and its early ending as a flight from his and his father's fears.

Christopher had labelled his own sexuality – whether gay or straight – as 'disordered'. I noted the word. It recurred time and again, and rang bells with me of a vocabulary of theological ethics. If I am not mistaken, it is the characteristic description of homosexuality in Roman Catholic moral theology.

He was afraid for his vocation, but clearly experienced his ministry as fulfilling and 'right'. He seemed to have a sense that he was in some way 'dangerous'. I found that inwardly I linked this with the dangers of both illicit and unsafe sexual encounter. I did not share this possible link, but kept it within me. I may have been wrong. Clearly though, Christopher identified strands of self-hatred in what he felt and did.

Christopher had learned a little T.A. as part of his theological education, and slipped into the jargon of T.A. of his own accord. This proved to be useful.

## Reflection

Christopher presented as overwhelmed by grief and shame. He was undermining his own beloved vocation. Christopher certainly struck me as someone who was acting upon some very self-destructive patterns. He saw himself as 'out of control'. As he talked with me, it became clearer that he meant both self-control and divine control.

The latter image seemed to me difficult as well as important. I recognized that I needed to keep close to what Christopher thought, believed and felt. For the therapist, particularly working in the area of faith – central, non-rational, truth-claiming faith – it is testing to hear accurately how another person puts together their world. Christopher and I may share a faith formally speaking, but I dare not even guess how much common ground we really have. This is a question of the client's frame of reference. Phenomenologically we assemble our worlds very differently. I wanted to avoid being seduced into feeling that I understood Christopher's world-view. What were the possibilities?

Divine control? He was out of control. My starting point within myself was to note that I do not see God as either controlling or 'in control'. Rather we live in a world in which there is freedom and pain (Worsley, 1996). Therefore, it is possible that Christopher and I simply hold to different theological views. However, I also note that God – whether or not He exists – is the recipient of human projections. Thus I regarded it as highly unlikely that Christopher's view of God would be wholly separate from his feelings about his own natural father. Perhaps, on these grounds, he wanted to be out of control, but his own father's control. In Freudian terms, this would be unresolved Oedipal material. I noted and bracketed off my thinking. I would need to listen more fully to Christopher.

I heard Christopher's grief and shame and guilt, all intermingled. Grief was found in sobbing. It was as if a part of him might have died. (What part? Would it be a goal of therapy for him to let go of this part, or to resurrect it? Again, listening.) Shame and guilt were both present. Each requires accurate attention. Guilt can come in a number of guises. For Christopher there was rational guilt, for he had transgressed his own code of ethical behaviour. It is important to be aware of the Rescuer within the counsellor who might want to 'save' the client from her own guilt. This is invasive. We all have a right to rational guilt, and to decide what constitutes it. Non-rational guilt – and I am aware that this very terminology is biased – is likely to be the product of our early acquired conditions of worth. What had Christopher ingested from his past about acceptability?

The difference between these two forms of guilt – they might be called moral and neurotic guilt – is not always easy to hear. The counsellor's frame of reference can certainly get in the way, particularly if I believe that no guilt is 'good'. I find a useful image in Fritz Perls' use of biting, chewing and digesting (Perls *et al.*, 1973, pp. 231–53). Perls taps into a basic act of human survival – eating. He distinguishes biting as a functional process, getting fed, from biting as aggression.

> **Personal Focus 6.1   Biting and introjection**
>
> Think of an apple. If you eat healthily and freely, there will be some pleasure in biting that is aggressive, for food needs to be killed. To eat freely is to chew and enjoy and experience, and then to swallow and fully assimilate the food, so that it is taken into the gut as effectively as possible. If an apple is force-fed, then the bite, compulsory, unavoidable, will be hard, vicious. The Other can be bitten through it. The piece of apple is swallowed nearly whole. It sticks, it hurts, it is thrown up or rots the gut. If I cannot escape being force-fed I will hurt someone. (It may be the Other or my Self.) This is introjection. This is the taking in of a hard and repulsive condition of worth.

I suggest that rational guilt is about applying freely to myself those standards which I have properly ingested. Non-rational guilt simply sticks in the throat.

Of course, life is not that simple. We have spent the latter part of our childhood, all of our adolescence and much of our adult life deciding what is ours and what is not, in terms of values and consequent guilt. We cannot finally know what belongs to us and what does not. It is decisional but rather approximate. Rightly or wrongly, Roman Catholicism is often seen as guilt-promoting. This is a stereotype. Yet, just to the extent that the Catholic culture does promote guilt, is the sincere and mature Catholic possessed by moral or neurotic guilt? Catholic friends of mine who know themselves well would hate to be too sure of the answer.

For Christopher, the boundaries between rational and non-rational guilt are yet to be established within our shared understanding of him.

Shame, by contrast with guilt, seems to me to have a primitive feel to it. I associate it with dream-experience, a standing naked in the middle of the road, for example. As I listened to Christopher, I became aware that his feelings of shame were ambivalent. He both dreaded being found out and longed to be found out. The feared secret incorporates the sought-after punishment that he felt his 'wicked' self so richly deserved.

Christopher's way of life was self-contradictory. He both aspired to a moral good – in his own terms – and seemed continually to undermine this aspiration in himself. He was what is often called 'acting out'. That is to say, his actions in the everyday world express his inner processes, his fears and fantasies. Thus I conjectured that his desire to risk illicit sex and his carelessness about safer sex were aspects of his self projected out onto the world. His actions allowed him to feel about himself in his interpersonal relationships exactly what he felt about himself internally and largely out of his own awareness – his self-concept.

Again, I want to use a psychodynamic concept to illuminate my own thinking about Christopher. Transference is the phenomenon whereby a past relationship (or even set of relationships) is lived out or created afresh in the present, so that present relationships become contaminated. Transference relationships happen when introjected feelings or conditions are 'acted out' in the present. Imagine for a moment walking into a room full of strangers, and feeling very insecure. One of my transference-habits will be to look for a person who reminds me of a familiar figure. 'You look like my Aunt Betty; she is really nice; that makes me feel better in the face of my insecurity.' In a similar way, it seemed to me that Christopher was living out some of his relationships as transferences from his past, while others looked to be genuine. As a rule of thumb, his genuine relationships fully valued the other person – much as he had been fully valued by his mother and his Church – while others used people instrumentally – much as he had been used by his father to fulfil his moral puritanism. Thus his sexual liaisons were not only 'disordered' (to use his own words and judgement), but were not aimed primarily at the sexual partner. Rather, I guessed, they were to defy his father. Yet to defy father was to risk self-destruction, and so Christopher built the potential for self-destruction through HIV into most of his liaisons. Thus a relationship that seemed to move towards intimacy rather than 'lust' had to be sabotaged.

The psychodynamic counsellor will classically foster such transferences within the therapeutic relationship, and then work with them, interpreting them to give the client insight. I did not do this with Christopher. As early as 1951, Rogers suggested that the problem with working with the transference is that it is slow and time-consuming (Rogers, 1951, p. 201). However, there are better reasons for not working in the classically psychodynamic way. Adopting the transference relationship within therapy in fact inhibits the therapist's genuineness. I do not want to overstate and thence polarize the two positions. Some parts of the psychodynamic tradition clearly see that the aim of therapy includes a genuine relationship between the client and the therapist (Guntrip, 1992). However, it is a cornerstone of person-centred work that genuineness is at the heart of therapy. Any fostering of the transference undermines the very rationale of person-centred work (Rogers, 1987). Yet for Christopher there is a problem. He lives out his transferences, his inauthentic self, with others, and not merely with me. What can I offer?

## Recognizing a Dilemma

In order to be fully in relationship with Christopher I had to be in touch with my own ambivalent feelings about him. Much of my internal process concerned my own counter-transferential feelings. I wanted to protect him not only from my disapproval, but also from my acceptance. My full acceptance of Christopher included engaging with his self-condemnation and with his self-destructive tendency, so as to feel as fully as possible what it was like to be that aspect of him without colluding with the acting out. To accept Christopher as he was before me was not only to refuse to judge or condemn, but also to refuse to take on board his self-condemnation. We were to spend a very considerable number of sessions simply living with his contradictory feelings and actions.

For me, the ego-state conceptualization of the way Christopher manifests his complex self-concept helps me maintain accurate contact with these tensions and ambivalences. Ego-state theory did two jobs in helping me to conceptualize Christopher acceptantly. It is fluent in describing the way Christopher lives out his conditions of worth interpersonally. It also allowed me to first express within myself my refusal to collude with his self-condemnation, and then to find a way of challenging this radical incongruence within him. How he spoke of his Child was not the way I felt about his Child.

## Conditions of Worth in Everyday Life

Conditions of worth have a basic structure to them. The worth of the individual is dependent upon them fulfilling the ONLY IF . . . set out by another. The other has an authority role towards the individual, sometimes as a parent, but often enough from within adult life. The individual's locus of personal evaluation has become exteriorized in the other. Particularly in the later years of his life, Carl Rogers explored the fact that society as a whole imposes conditions of worth (Rogers, 1978, chapters six and seven). It is not always clear where the conditions of worth which operate within any individual come from. The therapist must avoid jumping to conclusions.

In my work with Evelyn – see Chapter 4 – I was struck by the fact that she experienced her own needing as bad. I listened for weeks, expecting that eventually there would emerge a strong figure which would 'explain' this. I guessed that her father would be at the root of it. In the end, I offered her the comment that I could see no point of origin for her feeling that seeking the fulfilment of her needs was naughty. She was amazed that I had missed the point completely. It was Gerald. She had been reluctant to look at her relationship with Gerald. (Clients often feel that looking at current relationships is a breach of trust with that person.) Yet, she did not find it difficult to say that it was simply Gerald who could not accept her feelings. Her frustration was not a transference but a reasonable reaction to her partner's personality and behaviour. For Evelyn, one significant set of conditions of worth came from the present. She was only worthwhile and loveable if she did not ask for emotional attention! (I concede that she may have had from her past a particular valency for forming a relationship with a man like Gerald who denies her emotional need.)

Returning to Christopher, I am still uncertain about some aspects of his conditions of worth and self-concept. However, I estimate that he has internalized a number of sets of conditions of worth, which correspond to different structural elements in his personality. From his father, he might well have to cope with the following:

---

**Box 6.1 Christopher's likely conditions of worth**

- You are only acceptable if you are in control of your sexuality, and that means being continent and straight.
- You are only acceptable if you obey a set of external rules, and those are decided by the father.
- You are not tolerable – cannot be lived with – if you transgress.
- Obey rules and don't explore.
- If others – your sister – get it wrong, you are only acceptable if you stand out against them and become increasingly vigilant.
- You are only acceptable if you see yourself as sinful. (A double bind.)

---

From his mother, he would have felt more accepted. She was warmer. However, I note that one condition of worth would be that he was only acceptable to her as long as he did not 'make' her choose against her partner. Similarly, God and the Church, while each was experienced by him as accepting in varying degrees, also carried conditional elements. God is theologically 'Our Father'. Christopher seems to flout what he would see as God's will for him, much as I imagine he longed to find ways of flouting his own father's authority and oppression. Therefore, whatever the overt theology, God will likely have for him a darker side corresponding to his introjecting of his father's values. The Church certainly carries rule-like principles, which Christopher can flout and then judge himself against. The prohibition against a priest in particular committing fornication has a quality about it that resembles a condition of worth, just as long as Christopher refuses either to integrate the principle of celibacy into his own self or to reject it as not his.

Two quotations will help us to contact some of the qualities of Christopher's experience. The first is from Dave Mearns and Brian Thorne, the second from Thorne alone:

> Fortunately, the disapproval and rejection which many people experience is not such as to be totally annihilating. They are left with at least some shreds of self-esteem although these may often feel so fragile that the fear of final condemnation is never far away. It is as if such people are living according

to a kind of legal contract, and that they only have to put one foot wrong for the whole weight of the law to descend upon them.

(Mearns and Thorne, 1999, p. 8)

As a result of the overwhelming need for positive regard it is evident that for many people there develops over time a marked discrepancy between the self as perceived and the actual experience of the total organism. Where such a discrepancy exists Rogers speaks of an incongruence between self and experience. This incongruence leads to a psychological vulnerability which will often render the person anxious and confused whenever an experience is perceived or in some way anticipated as being incongruent with the structure of the self and the current self-concept.

(Thorne, 1992, p. 31)

Both of these quotations help me become more keenly aware of the ambivalences within Christopher. The first helps me symbolize inwardly the sense of condemnation which Christopher not only fears but paradoxically longs for. However, the element of legal contract is not simply an aspect of his self-concept which moves against his self-actualization. Christopher genuinely aspires to those values which threaten to condemn him. He is in breach of law-like rules which he also thoroughly assents to. It is as if Christopher has actualized two selves – a highly ethical self which is genuine enough, but which the over-hasty therapist might see as a moralized and moralizing false self, and a self which sees and rejects the very same principles which underlie the other self.

Christopher is split. He attempts with different parts of his awareness to put out into his world both versions of himself. His current relationships are governed by which version of himself is operative at the time.

The second quotation embodies a view of incongruence and the self-concept which is too simplistic for Christopher. He has at least two subsystems of the self, and each seems to act without regard for the other at this time. It is not the case that there is a self-concept and an 'actual experience of the whole organism'. Christopher's sub-personalities, his splitness, show that he runs at least two quite discrete self-concepts and experiences two separate sets of needs. The conflict between these two, what might be called a second-level incongruence, is then acted out as role and relationship conflict in Christopher's personal world.

## Ego-state Theory

For those not familiar with ego-state theory, I offer a brief summary. I refer in this section to the chart *Ego-State Theory: Crossing a Transaction* (Figure 6.1). The chart represents two individuals and a transaction between

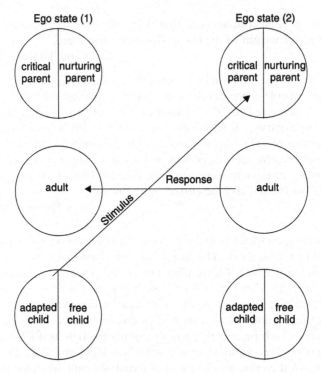

*Figure 6.1*   Ego-state theory: Crossing a transaction

them. A transaction is the expressing of a message in one direction (Stimulus) and the elicited reply (Response).

Each individual is seen as existing from moment to moment in one of three ego-states – the Parent, the Adult and the Child. The first and the third of these are subdivided into Critical Parent and Nurturing Parent, and Adapted Child and Free Child respectively.

The key point to grasp at all times is that this schema is strictly phenomenological. Thus we may talk about Christopher's Free Child or his Critical Parent. These ego-states stem from his experience. His Critical Parent and mine are therefore very different, just because we have had different experiences of being parented. This is a matter of overwhelming practical importance. I do not, I cannot, know what Christopher's Critical Parent is like; I have to discover through careful listening. In the past I have seen this schema likened to Sigmund Freud's three-part conceptualization of the person as Id, Ego and Superego. This could not be further from the truth. The contents and function of the Freudian Ego is a matter of theory; Christopher's Parent is knowable only by him. It is his phenomenon stemming from his own experience of being his parents' child. In grasping this point, we can see that to work with ego-state theory is compatible with other phenomenological approaches, and will need vigilant listening:

Berne saw transactional analysis as a 'systematic phenomenology' which could usefully fill a gap in psychological theory.... Berne's phenomenology concerned the description of ego states as phenomena which people experience subjectively and which he personally and clinically observed and intuited.

(Clarkson, 1992, p. 10)

The ego-states can be briefly summarized thus:

- *The Adult* is the individual responding in the here-and-now with all of her appropriate resources. The Adult corresponds closely to the organismic need of the person, although some organismic needs are met in other states. Note that some 'adult' activities are not from the Bernean Adult. For instance, sexual intimacy is perhaps best associated with the Free Child.
- *The Nurturing Parent* corresponds to those aspects of parenting activity that have been felt to be good, promoting growth, although perhaps fostering dependence as well. I recall offering help to a colleague. I took this to be either from my Adult or from some degree of Nurturing Parent. She responded with unusual and undue hostility. We were both amused, and on going over the transaction, I discovered that the offer of unsolicited help was, for her, Critical Parent, and would be met by the same. Again, the phenomenology of each of these states is specific to each person.
- *The Critical Parent* is the parental voice which either decrees behaviour or criticizes for behaviour or personal qualities. Care should be taken not to see the Nurturing Parent as 'good' and the Critical Parent as 'malign'. How these phenomena are experienced differs from person to person. I note that while my own children will resist my Critical Parent on the surface, they also seem to enjoy the security it gives when it sets acceptable boundaries.
- *The Adapted Child* state stems from those occasions when as a child we had to change our behaviour (and feelings?) in response to the adult world. Again, the Adapted and Free Child states can have negative and positive connotations.
- *The Free Child* incorporates a range of experience, from play to intimacy to rebellion. It is also closely related to the organismic need of the individual.

**Personal Focus 6.2   Identifying ego-states**

Think of a brief set of transactions with another person where you felt that there was real feeling attached to what was happening for you.

Write down the main exchanges between you.

Look at each exchange. Which ego-state do you sense was in play?

    Remember, ego-states can persist for a long while, but more usually they change from moment to moment.

    Are there any transactions that you feel unsure about? Review the brief definitions above or check the fuller ones in Stewart and Joines (1987). Trust your own feelings. The ego-states are your phenomena!

    Do particular states help you to recall or associate with memories of past relationships? What are the attached feelings?

There are two species of transactions. Complementary transactions – they would appear on the chart as parallel lines – tend to reinforce each other, and remain in operation over a sustained period of time. Crossed transactions tend to lead to a switch in ego-state, and bring about significant change in one or both parties.

A complementary transaction might happen between my bank manager and me in which we discussed my business needs in Adult, reaching a logical and mutually agreed solution to my questions. The payoff from this outcome would be, for me, that I got what I needed and that through rational nego-tiation, whereas his payoff would be an interview with a well-behaved and motivated customer, and a perception of himself as functioning well. By con-trast, I might have tried to appear to him as a Critical Parent, issuing the tacit threat that if I did not get what I needed then I would attack the bank's local reputation. He could reply from Adapted Child. My threat would have worked. The complementary transaction based on threat would continue.

However, in order to change another, it is necessary to cross the transaction. In the last example, the bank manager had at least three choices. He could have countered from his own Critical Parent and told me off for my moral blackmail. This can result in tears or a blazing row. He could have replied from Adult: 'Actually, that isn't how I do business.' He could have risked Free Child: 'You're all bluster, Richard, you old bugger. Let's have a scotch.'

These examples are always approximate. Look at the last reply. Is it Free Child or Nurturing or Critical Parent? I believe that it could be any of these. Which it is depends on the experience, the phenomenal field, of each of the participants. As with the example of my colleague above, confusion happens when we 'misdiagnose' each other's ego-states.

### Personal Focus 6.3  Crossing a transaction (1)

    Look again at the chart.

    See the crossed transaction, in which the first speaker (Stimulus) comes from Adapted Child, with the risk or desire to contact the other's Critical Parent.

> Note how the Responder crosses the transaction by coming from their Adult state in an attempt to shift the first speaker into Adult too.
> Can you illustrate this with two or three examples?
> What are the different possible outcomes/payoffs?

This is the crossed transaction in theory. How might it work in practice? Try to remain with responses to the client that are congruent with your normal way of therapy.

---

**Personal Focus 6.4   Crossing a transaction (2)**

> Very near to the beginning of a first counselling session, a client says, 'I want to warn you that I might try very hard to please you, and I'd like you to stop that happening.'
> What are the possible ego-states in play?
> How might the counsellor reply *unwisely*?
> What would be a desirable counsellor response? Why?

---

I want to end this section with a question for the reader about her practical self-awareness. In Chapter 2 (Personal Focus 2.2) I invited you to experiment with the notion of change of viewpoint. This related to the shift from classical to process perspectives in person-centred work. The above Personal Focuses are an opportunity to revisit this question. How does it feel to begin to conceptualize in ego-state theory terms? What are the opportunities? What are the resistances? How will you process each?

## Christopher's Ego-states

How does ego-state theory help the therapist? Conditions of worth are known and felt within the self. The self-concept is formed in the light of them. They are experienced as incongruent with the organismic needs of the whole self. Ego-state theory goes some way to describing how this incongruence manifests itself in interpersonal relationships.

My work with Christopher consisted of a thorough exploration between us of how he wanted to describe his current and past relationships. I was committed throughout to the person-centred stance that he, not I, was the expert on his frame of reference, his own phenomenology. This meant that I encouraged him to contact his 'felt sense' of each possible ego-state and to experiment with which felt authentically him (Gendlin, 1981, chapter one). The ego-state construct was available to both of us as a way of exploring Christopher's awareness, while remaining true to the power structure of a person-centred relationship.

The first figure to consider was Christopher's relationship with his father. Clearly he experienced father as controlling and mother as nurturing on most occasions. He could make more sense of his defensive activity as a child who tried to please father both through his natural humour and through much-resented obedience. He could identify his need to find his father's love. His mother did not make up for this. The concept of crossing a transaction made it clear to Christopher that he could at least consider whether there were new patterns of relating available between him and his now-ageing father. Yet he does not at the moment hold out much hope.

Christopher wrestles with his own morality and his guilt at his behaviour. He recognizes that the problem is not about fornication *tout court*, but rather about his object-like sense of his partners, particularly when they seek true intimacy with him. He began to sense that they were objects rather than people just to the extent that they were pawns in a game with his father. The nature of that game puzzled us both for a while.

Guilt became more clearly focused when Christopher explored the possibility of being able to decide which ego-state he chose to act out of. He saw that his Adapted Child was not the only possibility. (His anger and his self-destructive urge had blinded him to this. He felt compelled to rebel or conform.) He began to experiment inwardly with the possibility of acting from Adult.

I felt uneasy with this. It seemed such an effort, as though he had to perform adequately, was a condition of worth. This contrasted with his felt-sense of the role of Nurturing Parent, the living out of a thoroughly digested gift from mother, I guessed. His ministry with others was richly imbued with this quality, both Nurturing and Parent. My feeling was that the former was good, the latter a little patronizing. As he grows in self-esteem, maybe he will find it within him to be less parental with his congregation. I have no desire to share that insight with him! He will probably get there without even being aware of it.

Gradually, Christopher began to develop an awareness of two *personae* working in his past. In his teenage years, he saw himself as having to survive by constraining his Adaptive/Rebellious Child with quite a bit of Adult. His self-concept was of a rational, aware human being who, because of pressure from his persecuting father, had to work very hard to contain the disruptive Child within.

I recall the vividness of the moment when I blurted out: 'I am not sure I believe that story any more.' I do not normally challenge so insensitively. I was...well, angry. I knew I was defending something worthwhile, but it took me a while to get to what it was.

'You keep telling me how difficult your Child is and how hard you have to work to contain it. I can feel the burden on you. It is an immense weight. It was like that when you lived at home and it is still like that in the face of what you call your temptations. Its just that I want to protest. Your Child isn't like that. That is your Father's version of it. I'm wondering if that *really* is your version.' Twenty-three sessions into therapy, it just about felt OK to take that sort of risk.

Christopher looked stunned, pole-axed. For 40 minutes he worked through my challenge. The outcome was that he came to see a mischievous, playful, loveable and, above all, sexually alive Free Child. He is now left with the conviction that the Free Child deserves his own attention – the core conditions – and some room to play. Whatever decision he makes about sex and celibacy, maybe he and I can stop talking about fornication in a po-faced way!

# Being Person-Centred?

In his recent book, *Person-Centred Therapy: A Revolutionary Paradigm*, Jerold Bozarth (1998) discusses the particularly American issue of whether a person-centred counsellor can use a battery of psychological tests with a client. He concludes, 'The conditions for the use of tests are that they are used within the framework of the therapist's dedication to the client's world and "self-authority"' (Bozarth, 1998, p. 128). What is true of such a tool-like object as a test is even truer of conceptual frameworks like ego-state theory. When using ego-state theory, these questions are important:

---

**Personal Focus 6.5   Am I being person-centred?**

- How far on is the relationship? If it is not well developed and mature, why should you want to risk using a tool, potentially a trick of the trade? Be aware of your motivation.
- Are the core conditions thoroughly in place? What in detail is your evidence for your answer?
- How do you see the use of ego-states? Listen to yourself. Does it speak to you of your expertise? If so, what are you going to do about this?
- How will the client see it? Even if you are clear within yourself, the client will not necessarily share your view. The power relationship within therapy needs constant vigilance. If in doubt, deal with it openly and congruently. Ask.
- Consult your supervisor about pay-offs for you. Will the use of ego-state theory 'unstick' a stuck client? Why do you want to unstick your client? What is wrong with being stuck?

> Have you been asked or do you offer? Know why, for you, this matters.
> Above all, have you made a sub-contract to facilitate the work?

## Into Practice

Personal Focus 6.5 sets out some useful warnings about how to get it right or wrong. Yet, beneath the everyday wisdom is a deeper issue. Christopher, like a number of clergy whom I see, had already come across a number of T.A. concepts. To use these is simply to be willing to talk the client's language. However, unlike Jerold Bozarth, who argues that it is important that a client *asks* for a psychological test, I sometimes teach one or another client to use it. It is no more than expanding the client's vocabulary. But which concept and why?

Clients process in particular ways. I am struck by the fact that some clients make progress without ever conceptualizing their inner state, their conditions of worth or whatever. Other clients have a valency for thinking it through and needing to know. Clients process differently.

Christopher, however much he needed to have his torrent of emotion heard, was, after a while, in need of considering his inner possibilities and developing what I have come to see as an appropriate style of psychological wisdom. For him, ego-state theory fitted his own processing. He did it like that. The deep skill and empathy is to listen long enough to a client to intuit how they process their material. Be aware of how the client needs to process.

Ego-state theory in use combines an active cognitive element – thinking in depth and in full awareness – with the ability to contact a felt-sense of the rightness for them of constructs. That was Christopher's way of being, of processing. Others will have different needs. Some will need to have more immediate access to their own bodily awareness. We will speak of them in the next chapter.

Ego-state theory can represent elements of the client's inner processing. As such, it is a useful conceptualization which can aid the therapist in empathy and the client in reflexivity.

## Further Reading

Berne, E. (1964) *Games People Play: The Psychology of Human Nature*. Harmondsworth, Penguin.
Harris, T.A. (2004) *I'm OK – You're OK*. London, Harper Collins.

Both of these are popular psychology – an art form in which T.A. excels. They are both worth the read. *Games People Play* may sound an old book, but do not be fooled. It is still in print and worth the read. Parties will never be the same again!

Clarkson, P. (1992) *Transactional Analysis Psychotherapy: An Integrative Approach.* London, Routledge.

One of the most scholarly and complete accounts of T.A. therapy. Excellent reference book, but tough to read from cover to cover.

Stewart, I. and V. Joines (1987) *T.A. Today.* Nottingham, Lifespace.

A very lively, popular and yet accurate introduction to T.A. A useful guide for student, practitioner and counselling tutor alike.

# 7

# Mirrors of Our Being: A Person-Centred Use of Gestalt Theory

Gestalt therapy challenges us to see that the client's frame of reference includes all of her awareness, both that which is within her reflexive consciousness and that which is at the very edge of her awareness. Gestalt has a particular genius for describing this so as to give full emphasis to the body, to bodily experience and to its interruption. In acknowledging this emphasis, I am abiding by the principle of the Chicago position statement that person-centred therapy is holistic. No aspect of the frame of reference of the client can be ignored. Classical client-centred therapy runs the risk of ignoring the somatic aspect, embodied awareness.

The chapter revisits Rennie's (1998) idea of metacommunication, but this time taking metacommunication as addressing a level of awareness that is embodied in the counselling relationship but is usually at the edge of awareness. Understanding the client's embodied awareness is then addressed as an aspect of empathy, and linked to Carl Rogers' notion of the fully functioning person. Finally, there is a detailed exploration of the key conceptual tool, the Gestalt cycle of awareness, which leads to a consideration of the use of this in person-centred practice. This bridging to practice includes the case of David, a study of a piece of supervision.

## Awareness as an Aspect of the Client's Frame of Reference

Early on in a first counselling session, a client says, 'I want to warn you that I might try very hard to please you, and I'd like you to stop that happening.'

Her voice is small and plaintive. She uses her Adult inadvertently to reinforce her Adapted Child state. Paradoxically, the very desire to escape from an ego-state, and the underlying recognition that this is where she is, comes to be expressed in terms of the very ego-state that she longs to escape. I notice from this that neither a making conscious of conditions of worth nor of ego-states nor of any other useful enough construct turns out to be necessary for the client to change. Phenomenological exploration seems to go deeper than merely making conscious underlying mechanisms. The person-centred therapist is committed to working at experiential depth. This means escaping head knowledge as the main source of change.

I am conscious of at least two possible responses to the client's statement. I believe that the conventional person-centred response, particularly at this early stage, would be to reflect the client's underlying feeling:

I guess you feel that you don't want to slip into an old pattern of pleasing and want me to help you avoid it.

However, I much prefer a more experiential alternative:

You don't want to end up trying to please me. Perhaps that is an old pattern for you that you know well. Yet, you want me to stop you doing it. I guess I'm not going to give in to that one *(said with chuckle)*. I reckon that if you want to avoid that trap you can do that by yourself without me pointing it out to you.

What is the difference between these two responses?

First I do not see either as right. I prefer the second. It would be arrogant to call it better than the first. Therapists have to work at the level and in the way that is theirs, and with which they are at ease. I feel as much at ease with the second as the first.

The first response acknowledges the feelings of the client and as such is an accurate and empathic grasp of the client's conscious thinking and feeling. It has the great virtue of allowing the client a lot of space to hear what they have said and to work with it. I acknowledge that the second response takes away some of this freedom to hear the conscious content and to reflect on it.

The second response is for me a more deeply congruent reaction to the client's whole frame of reference, both that which she knows she is saying and that which is implicit and at the edge of her awareness. It reflects far more accurately the client's paradoxical process: even when I want to escape Adapted Child I end up doing it from Adapted Child.

Is the second response more interpretative? Well, it could be. Interpretation is not a discrete action that I can always recognize as such. It is an action *within a relationship*. To interpret is to inform the client of a meaning, and thus to be powerful. To explore is to be puzzled together. For me, the second response is not interpretative, just because it is a risk, a setting out to explore whether my way of responding is empathic or crass. If the client can say, 'OK, thanks for that. I'll try and trust myself more', then it was empathic. If the client feels a little unheard or even rejected, then it was crass. The second response to the client has two qualities to which I want to draw attention. The first is that it is striving for empathy that draws the client to discover feelings and experiences nearer to the edge of her awareness.

The second quality of the response is subtle, but important. It is to be the subject of this chapter. The response is, I believe, more in tune with the whole of the client's awareness. Awareness is not to be confused with consciousness or self-consciousness. I do not mean by it the sort of awareness that is described by the sentence: 'I am now aware that...'. What I point to is that sort of awareness when the whole person, the whole organism, is aware. Some of the things I am aware of are out of my consciousness. For instance, I find that I am tapping my foot. I look at it. Yes, of course! I am *so* bored. It is as if my foot were more aware of my boredom than my censored and controlled, conditioned and well-behaved conscious mind.

For my client, she was conscious of her need to put to rest her condition of worth. In fact she would try hard to please me by trying not to please me! Her larger awareness knew the paradox of this. Knowing where she wanted to go was not enough. Therefore she also communicated her stuckness in this through the mannerisms of the Adapted Child. She invited me to respond not to an Adult request but to her stuckness in Adapted Child.

This is another example of the fact that we live upon a continuum between reflexivity and spontaneity. The reflexive element in my client knew her own conditions of worth. However, only the immediate and spontaneous element in her could communicate her stuckness in Adapted Child. It is as if her conditions of worth have a built-in self-preservation system. They not only say, 'make sure that you please others!' They add, 'and if you ever spot this, make sure that you confront it in a way that still pleases others'.

I recognize an annoying quirk of language here. Awareness has two almost contradictory meanings, and I need both. The word can mean conscious awareness, particularly in the phrase 'edge of awareness' that person-centred practitioners prefer over talking of the unconscious, with all of its Freudian baggage. It also means the awareness of the whole organism. In short, some forms of awareness (sense two) are out of awareness (sense one).

Yet this is not just a linguistic matter. We need to make up our minds what we mean by a client's frame of reference. Is it really just what they think and feel at the moment? I believe not. It includes all that they have within them, their full awareness, whether or not in their consciousness at any particular point of time. My client's conscious desire to please is no more a part of her frame of reference than her stuckness in escaping her Adapted Child. Of course, those thoughts and feelings which are fully conscious to the client are easier to check out. Nor can we be crass with the other elements of awareness. They have to be explored with care and humility. But both elements are aspects of the client's frame of reference. A frame of reference, a view of the world, is made up of the reactions and tendencies of the whole organism.

When the whole person is addressed within the person-centred relationship, when all aspects of client awareness (in the wider sense) are accorded the core conditions, the client may more readily find within herself the resources to make the changes described by Rogers (1957c):

> The self becomes increasingly simply the subjective and reflexive awareness of experiencing. The self is much less frequently a perceived object, and much more frequently something confidently felt in process.
>
> (p. 153)

## Expressing Our Organismic Need: A Gestalt Perspective

In 1951, Fritz Perls wrote:

> Experience occurs at the boundary between the organism and its environment...Experience is the function of this boundary, and psychologically what is real are the whole configurations of this functioning, some meaning being achieved, some action completed...We speak of the organism contacting the environment, but it is the contact that is the simplest and first reality.
>
> (Perls *et al.*, 1973, p. 273)

Perls' approach to therapy does justice to the wholeness and irreducibility of the human being. We are not just minds but a complete system including as much the body as the mind. The unconscious is not merely the suppressed part of the mind – as it is with Freud – but includes those aspects of bodily existence which are very much present as 'mindedness', yet out of awareness (sense one). Thus my mind can express itself as much in the fidgeting of my foot or the fist-making of my hand, or in the breathlessness of my asthma as in my thoughts and feelings. (See Bateson, 1973, for a systemic account of mindedness.)

How I am, my frame of reference, the whole way I relate to the world and my environment, expresses itself through my body as much as through my thinking or feeling. All contact between my self and my environment is an expression of who I am. The holistic view of the self which is to be found in Gestalt thinking corresponds well with Rogers' view of the organismic self, that part of the self which, often out of awareness and overlain with our dysfunctional self-concepts, strives to actualize itself. The imagery that Rogers has for this part of the self is closely allied to Perls' thinking:

> The actualizing tendency can of course be thwarted, but it cannot be destroyed without destroying the organism. I remember that in my boyhood the potato bin in which we stored our winter supply of potatoes

was in the basement, several feet below a small basement window. The conditions were unfavourable but the potatoes would begin to sprout.

(Rogers, 1978, p. 8)

We as people are analogous to potatoes (in spite of very obvious differences) to the extent that we both strive to fulfil our needs in relationship to our surrounding environment.

Transactional Analysis helps us describe phenomenologically the ways we have of contacting our environment interpersonally. Gestalt thinking helps us describe the ways our selves behave, often at the very edge of our awareness, so as to express our organismic needs. I prefer the second response to my client proposed above because it addresses more holistically the client's process. That process goes beyond what she thinks and feels. It is embodied in her relating to me. When I address this relating – when I am congruent about our shared way of being, our shared frame of reference – I open up for both of us new ways of being together.

## Awareness and Metacommunication

It is characteristic of a process-orientated or experientially orientated way of working within the person-centred approach that the therapist and client together will be open to self-talk, to relational-talk – what Rennie calls metacommunication (Rennie, 1998, chapter eight).

> By paying close attention to context, to the manner and tone which the client says things, to the gestures given, to what is not said as well as what is said and to the client's body language, the person in the role of counsellor empathetically seeks to understand the one in the role of client and, correspondingly, to stimulate her to achieve greater self-understanding.
>
> (Rennie, 1998, p. 89)

Rennie then points to four forms or purposes of metacommunication (Rennie, 1998, p. 98):

---

**Box 7.1   Four forms of metacommunication**

- the therapist reveals the purposes of her own communication.
- the therapist reveals the impact of the client's communication.
- the therapist enquires into the purposes behind the client's communication.
- the therapist enquires into the impact on the client of the therapist's own communication.

---

Metacommunication should be used sparingly, for it is indeed beyond communication, and, like other forms of therapist-congruent communication, moves the client away from her own frame of reference for the time being.

In spite of this risk, metacommunication addresses the client's whole being and her relationship with the therapist, with a new level of questing for understanding with deeper empathy. The knack is to keep the interpersonal process feeling empathic. Metacommunication should always be aimed at conveying a deepen-ing desire to understand the client. A fairly common example of metacommunication might be exemplified in my work with Roberta:

---

### Box 7.2   Metacommunication – an example

*Roberta*: When I was driving here this afternoon, wondering what I was going to talk about, I really had no idea that I was going to talk about my sex life.

*Richard*: It's a struggle to talk about it. (Pause) And I notice that you've brought it to a male therapist.

---

The second part of what I said revealed not a cold observation but a sense of the impact that Roberta's work had on me. How remarkable that she chooses to work with me in this area! Behind this are a number of questions that she might then raise for herself. Is she comfortable enough to work with me on this? Does she want to move to another area of work? Is it important that I am male to her? If so, why? This exchange opens up her awareness of the context and purposes of her work. If she is taking a risk, what is it that is trying to actualize itself?

Roberta used my intervention to explore what she wanted. She came to the conclusion that her mother would have expected her to have put up with a lack of sexual satisfaction, as though she were not worthy of it. She wanted to protest that, at long last, she was willing to take the risk of setting her face against this script. My maleness increased the immediate risk. In feeling the risk she also felt her newly discovered determination to affirm herself in what she dared to ask for.

---

### Box 7.3   Exploring metacommunication

Take each of Rennie's four types of metacommunication in turn. Remember that his way of describing metacommunication is neither the only one nor is it complete.

---

For each type, devise an example either in your imagination or from your own case work.

What effects do you imagine that the metacommunication might have?

What could be its benefits?

What could be its shortcomings?

Above all, how would you feel saying what you have just devised? It is important to be at home in all forms of communication, and above all to be using what you are doing to facilitate your client in a relationship in which the power dynamics are non-abusive, and in which the core conditions are embodied.

Very occasionally, I find myself using metacommunicative exchanges on a larger scale. I return to the case of Evelyn in Chapters 4 and 5. Evelyn spent quite a while working with me on her relationship with her immediate boss. She came to understand how her relationship with her parents deeply influenced her adult relationships. She reached a point in which she could say, 'Here I go again. This is not how I want to react.'

On one occasion, she went back into school. Her boss was by any stretch of the imagination unreasonable with her. I found myself almost stopping the listening process to protest that I just felt so angry with him. I then used some of my supervisor's skills to explore why I felt angry in particular. What had he done?

The benefit for Evelyn was that she then explored her surprise and delight at my anger. She had experienced herself as growing away from not seeing why communications went wrong for her, towards seeing that sometimes she might misconstrue what was being said to her at the emotional level. The result was that she missed the fact that some problems were just other people being very difficult.

This was useful work for her to have done, but I was also aware of the possible problems of reacting in this way. First, it was an implementation of my own judgement about her and her boss. I would normally want to keep my judgements, even in the sense of estimations, out of my listening. Secondly, it could have been, or be felt to be, collusive: I am on your side – isn't he a bastard! Thirdly, it did interrupt the flow of her thinking. I made the judgement that this was worthwhile. (This judgement is always necessary for therapists' expression of their own congruence.) Yet I must admit that I have no idea whether she would have got to the same place completely by herself. Fourthly, I might have been acting out of my own desire to rescue my client.

Metacommunication is not easy. It carries risks. In assessing these risks I need to have a clear notion that whatever I do takes place in a relationship which embodies and expresses the core conditions of therapy. I can interrupt my client with my strong responses only because I rarely do that.

Metacommunication addresses the processes between therapist and client and within the client. It is one way only of practising awareness. All acts of awareness are mirrors to our Being.

## Awareness and its Edge: A Study in Empathy with Process

Alistair, whose narrative was a part of Chapter 5, is a very competent pianist. Towards the end of his work with me, he told me that at those times when he felt a low-level, gnawing depression, he was unable to play the piano. I think that I would have taken scant note of this, taking it for granted as typical of depression. However, Alistair was keen to work on this. He felt increasingly that it stood for something important. I thought again of Rogers (1957c): 'Internal communication is clear with feelings and symbols well matched' (Rogers, 1957c, p. 154). Alistair's persistent fascination with the figure of 'not playing the piano' suggested to me that his process was striving to symbolize a need to grasp experientially an aspect of his own experience of being depressed.

I am truly intrigued and often moved by clients' ability to know at the edge of their awareness what their own needs are and to strive to fulfil them. Alistair sought meaning in an experience which he clearly felt to be an embodiment of... what? We both needed to spend time being puzzled.

The phenomenological method as put forward by both Rogers and Perls is a constant reminder to listen for those times when we need to pay careful attention with our clients to their experience and awareness. Their frames of reference comprise more than content and feelings. Alistair and I agreed that we would pursue what he was experiencing throughout a complete session.

Exploring an experience in detail in many ways resembles day-to-day person-centred therapy, except for the fact that, if the client seems to want to focus upon this exploration, then I usually make a very brief subcontract to share in that task until the client feels it is in some way completed. At heart, this is an undertaking on my part to remain persistently with that exploration. I will be far less willing to follow a client into other territory, because we have agreed to undertake a specific task together. I note that such exploration has a sense of phenomenological research to it. As such, I doubt that I would undertake it with a disturbed or very distressed client. It belongs to the latter part of therapy, where improved function in the client leads to increased curiosity and desire to learn from experiential reflection. I have to be wary of undue steering of the client through questioning. Questions have their place especially in this phenomenological exploration, but I need to spend as much time as possible reflecting in detail what it is I experience the client as saying and feeling.

I asked Alistair to imagine what it is like to try and play while feeling depressed. I had no sense of him simply feeling too down to bother. Not playing felt active. He was interrupting himself from taking up an otherwise pleasurable activity. As I imagined him playing, I reflected to him my awareness that he approached much of his music as well-crafted, beautiful, but with occasional pleasure in the cacophonous. The latter he could relate to anger or rebellion. When he was depressed, he had trouble accessing his anger. This is not surprising, but nor is it the full story.

The notion of well-crafted beauty threw him back to talking of his childhood. All the while this seemed to me connected to the physiological experience of interruption. His parental home was 'loving, God-fearing but not prone to joy'. Well-crafted beauty would not be welcomed there. There was a puritanical harshness to that environment.

The image or symbol of not playing the piano, he explained to me, seemed to be about how difficult it is to feel well-crafted beauty when depressed. This in turn resonated with his lack of motivation to take care of himself at such times, and inversely with his new-found ability to assert his practical need for self-care in his work and his family life.

When Alistair is depressed, it is not that he does not play the piano. It turns out, I learned from him, that he interrupts his desire to play, in order to symbolize his lack of willingness to care for himself. He mobilizes his musical self and then blocks any acting upon it. Far from being lethargic, muscularly atonic, he is tense, blocking, self-withholding.

The next stage of his work was to return to his increased felt-need to care for himself. For Alistair, this means claiming a mental right to space for himself, and implementing this self-consciously through work-a-day strategies of time management.

## Awareness and Being Fully Functioning

Fritz Perls developed the notion that we experience life in one of three zones (Houston, 1990; Sills *et al.*, 1995). The inner zone is composed of bodily sensations and feelings; the outer zone, the world as experienced through the five senses, the modes of contact; the middle zone is made up of images and phantasies which strictly speaking are part of our inner life but in fact seem to refer to the environment in which we live.

Healthy living is for Perls about making good contact with the environment. This enables us to complete experiential Gestalts just as the organism needs:

From the point of view of psychotherapy, when there is good contact – e.g., a clear, bright figure freely energized from an empty background – then there is no peculiar problem concerning the relations of 'mind' and 'body' or 'self' and 'external world'.

(Perls *et al.*, 1973, p. 303)

When Alistair played the piano fluently, that act was for him a bright figure. The background receded. It was (re)creation. He was renewed as his playing refreshed him from that which he could relegate to the dull greyness of the margins of awareness. When he blocked this playing far from seeming apathetic, he was tense and self-denying:

we have here the typical picture of neurosis: *under-aware proprioception and finally perception, and hypertonus of deliberateness and muscularity*. (Yet let us insist again that this condition is not unfunctional, in the given chronic low-grade emergency.)

(Perls *et al.*, 1973, p. 313)

Perls makes two points here. The first is that, under what he terms neurotic stress, a person will be unduly unaware of the inner zone and will not perceive and therefore understand this lack of awareness. This is accompanied by stiffness of action and muscular tension. (Alistair was too tense to be merely apathetic.) However, Perls also makes the point that this condition is not a dysfunction in the sense of a meaningless going-wrong of awareness. It carries other information. If Alistair had been in danger, then this focus upon a tense being and a resistance to playing would have been appropriate. He was interrupting his playing just because he felt a danger that existed, not in the outer zone, the material world, but within his middle zone. He interrupted himself just when he was most keenly aware of the lack of self-care he had, and associated with his birth-home.

As we complete each Gestalt of our experiencing, we permit ourselves to move through a cycle of experience without undue interruption. This cycle Alistair was denying to himself. Gestalt theory describes the cycle and its interruptions in details.

---

**Personal Focus 7.1   Awareness and the flow of experience**

- In a quiet room, find a position in which you can happily relax. I find being flat on my back on a semi-firm surface works best for me.
- Give yourself mental permission to escape the day's concerns.
- Close your eyes and become aware of your proprioceptive sensing. Be aware of the pressure of your clothes, of the surface below

you, of your limbs as they touch each other and above all of the internal sensations of each part of your body.

As you relax, some part of you will 'stand out' as a clear figure. Note it and pay it attention from within. It will probably soon change. Do not either make this happen or block it. Simply note what happens.

You are likely to 'move around' your body in a fairly random way, with each proprioceptive figure forming against the ground of your general awareness and then fading and giving way to another figure.

Note how it is likely that there is a deepening of relaxation as proprioceptive Gestalten are allowed freely to complete. I find this a remarkably effective relaxation exercise.

Enjoy.

## The Cycle of Experience

The diagram *The Gestalt cycle of experience* (Figure 7.1) summarizes the pattern of a complete Gestalt. It is not the purpose of this chapter to discuss the cycle in detail; such material can be found elsewhere (Sills *et al.*, 1995; Harris, 2003). I will use the diagram to describe Alistair's pattern, and then look at the way an understanding of this concept can be of use to the person-centred therapist. Before this, however always, it is useful to check out the contents of the diagram against real experience.

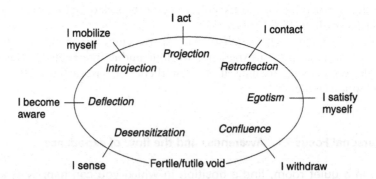

*Figure 7.1*  The Gestalt cycle of experience. The ellipse represents the boundary between self and environment. On the outside of the cycle are stages of experiences, while on the inside are the modes of self-interrupt which correspond to each stage of the cycle

**Personal Focus 7.2   Tangerine Gestalt**

Find a wholesome and appetizing tangerine – if you like them.

Eat it.

Note in as much detail as possible how you do this, both in terms of the sequence of events and the sensations and feelings which accompany this.

Check this out against the outer circle of stages of the cycle on the diagram.

Did you interrupt your own experiencing. How? When? Does the inner circle of interruptions help you understand this at all?

The interruptions may be unfamiliar to you. Remember that any interruption can be functional as well as dysfunctional. If we could not interrupt our experience, fire alarms would be useless. Spend time thinking about the meaning of each interruption. The first four should be the more familiar. I desensitize when I 'choose' not even to begin to feel something. I deflect when I actively prefer some other awareness. I introject when I swallow whole a piece of experience, in particular those introjects that then become life-scripts for me. I project when I put out onto others what I might do myself.

Retroflection is the turning back upon myself of an action, so that I do for myself what I want others to do for me. Thus I retroflect when, feeling the need for comfort, I stroke my own arm. In fact, I would prefer someone else to do this. Egotism – not the vice of being self-centred, by the way – is the act of commentating to oneself upon an action. Egotism uses enforced reflexivity to deprive me of spontaneous, full experiencing. Confluence happens when I become unable to distinguish between myself and another. I notice that sometimes I refer in conversation to my partner and I as 'we', without even consulting her. I habitually do not note that we are separate human beings. It angers her, of course.

The diagram associates each interruption with a particular phase of the cycle. There is some truth in this affinity, but it is partial. Any interruption can happen at any stage in the cycle. Explore this for yourself. Select a stage of the cycle, and then an interruption other than the one tied to it. See if you can devise a piece of experiencing whereby this interruption would cut through this particular stage of the cycle.

When I did the tangerine exercise recently, I noted the following results for me:

### Box 7.4   Me and my tangerine

- Almost before I thought that I had begun, I had got in touch with the texture of the skin – cool, pitted, smooth and yet uneven, soft, pliable, loose. And with a smell, not orange, more perfumed. **I SENSE**.
- I note these sensations. I can do this briefly, non-verbally, naturally. Or I can recite them to myself. Spontaneous or reflexive. **I AM AWARE**.
- My jaw and tongue become a figure for me. Not very clearly, but a sort of physical apprehension. Strangely, it reminds me of sexual excitement. I salivate. I am teeth. **I MOBILIZE MYSELF**.
- I open the tangerine, examining the contents – a cycle within a cycle – and then take a segment and put it in my mouth. It dawns on me that I have become aware of the softness of the skin of the segment – another mini-cycle – and then I crush it between tongue and palate. **I ACT**.
- The juice is cold and sharp and wonderful. It contrasts with the smoothness – almost warmth – of the segment skin. **I MAKE FINAL CONTACT**.
- Each segment consumed, and each enjoyed, I feel the goodness of the whole act for me. **I SATISFY MYSELF**.
- Gradually, the act of eating the tangerine subsides again into the background. I feel like washing my slightly sticky hands now. I rest for a few moments, but before I have chance to get up, someone speaks to me . . . **I WITHDRAW**.

## Into Practice

How does the construct of the cycle of experience help me to work with Alistair?

First, I avoid using it diagnostically. Person-Centred practitioners do not diagnose. They offer a relationship. However, I remember being hooked on one client's experience. I noted late on in therapy that she could not make a clear, bright figure. Other things swamped her. She could not concentrate. As we explored these sensations, I became convinced that she had an awareness deficit and I inwardly likened it to being dyslexic. I asked a colleague for a few minutes supervision. He is an experienced Gestaltist. Very quickly he moved me away from this diagnostic frame of mind to remind me that all interrupted experience is likely to be an expression of meaning – unless there is an organic cause like a brain lesion.

I returned to my client. She was quite easily able to discover within herself a parallel to her interruption – the heavy demands made upon her as a doctoral student, with a constant fear of wasting time, money and esteem. Undue pleasure must be stopped!

An interruption is very often the expression of a condition of worth or some similar introject. I have discovered that a careful phenomenological description of the experience and its interruption will facilitate the client in contacting the meaning-for-her. I can neither interpret nor diagnose.

With Alistair, I notice that he interrupts his mobilization before he plays. He allows himself to feel the need to play – otherwise there would be a far vaguer sense of 'never getting round to it'. He stops himself playing. I can get in touch with the possibility of at least three of the seven interruptions having some meaning in Alistair's case. While he clearly does not desensitize himself – he can feel at the edge of awareness that he might need or want to play – he deflects at least some of the force of this: I am down, and it's not worth it. He focuses on the bad feelings. He is stopped because of past introjection. He has swallowed down whole the message that life should not be enjoyed vibrantly. While in much of his adult life he has fought against and disowned this script, when he feels depressed he moves back into the sense that joy is forbidden to him and that creativity and structured beauty are not right. While deflection and introjection are important interruptions, so too is retroflection, but rather by anticipation.

When Alistair is well and plays well he is spontaneous and alive and outward-focused. To play for comfort would be too painful, I imagine. It would be like a loss of vivid spontaneity in favour of a sensation akin to self-pity: I no longer play, I just console myself.

To understand how all of this helps me in my work with Alistair, I need to return to the concept of the client's frame of reference. I seek to understand him as fully as possible. This includes the elements of his being which are at the edge of his own awareness. At the simplest, when I note that Alistair's self-interruption is not just 'what depressed people do', but has meaning, this prevents me from ignoring this part of his experience. I focus on it. It interests me. I listen. Perhaps he too will focus on it if I can listen carefully.

Theory does not tell me how the client is. It suggests to me new ways of imagining and talking with myself about his experience. It is one aspect – and only one – of my striving for empathy. When I can formulate with care in my thinking what might be happening for Alistair, just as when I listen and feel with him, the theory can become a mirror of his Being.

## Bridging

Because what is within our awareness (sense one) is only a part of our frame of reference, then many activities that can be undertaken with clients and supervisees in a person-centred way can help the person express what is there without the interruptiveness of the reflexive. I mean this. A client talks of his boss and protests that they get on fine. He really likes the man. All the while his right foot swings to and fro. A Gestalt therapist might invite the man to exaggerate this. It becomes a fully formed kick. Does it mean anything? The man is suddenly fully aware of his suppressed desire to kick his boss where the pain would be worst. This activity of helping the client relate a piece of behaviour to its meaning is known as bridging (Silverstone, 1997, pp. 21–5). Note that it differs from interpretation. The therapist does not tell or even suggest the meaning, but invites the client to observe and comment. The task of the therapist is only to notice and thus to encourage the client's meaning to appear.

Bridging is bound to be directive in at least the sense that the therapist identifies a phenomenon as of interest to herself. She is likely to direct the attention of the client to that phenomenon. Some person-centred or experiential therapists might be happy to undertake the above experiment with the kicking action. This is both directive and directorial. Others might only want to use the bridging as a basis for understanding, for empathy. A typical example of this sort of bridging would be Carl Rogers' comment to Kathy that he can see sadness in her moistening eyes. Any focused empathy is directive, and any empathy which takes as its cue the client's process is a bridging movement.

By way of example, a moment from supervising David:

## Case 7.1   David

David is an able therapist, some three years post-Diploma. He is intelligent, articulate, at times verbose. I longed to get him to be freer to contact his clients' material. One day, I suggested tentatively that we try to look at a case non-verbally. I didn't know the case at all. He asked to work with stones. I handed him a box of stones, and expected him to take them out onto the table. Instead, he put the box on the floor, and we gathered round and looked from above. He looked but did not touch. This was not like him. He is very 'hands-on'. After a while he suggested that one stone reminded him of his client, others in the box did not stand out for him. A number of stones began to form into a Gestalt, a pattern which made them separate from their neighbours. These stones, their appearance, texture, colour, position had become for him the client and her family. He was puzzled. He looked from all angles. The activity consumed 40 minutes! I reflected to him what I saw, and what he said. I tried to get close to his feelings about this family.

He did not touch. 'No,' he replied, 'and it feels like that with my work. I listen but I do not touch.'

The client touched parts of all the other disparate stones which formed the network of her family. She could not be moved. 'If I touch her, I will disturb everything, and you can't do that.'

David had felt within himself a real apprehension lest therapy be effective and move the client to change. Maybe change would be difficult, even in a sense disastrous. But it was up to the client to choose, and not up to David to keep her safe by subverting the process.

His work with her became freer, more focused and more congruent. The stones, together with my bridging, had embodied his unaware awareness as a mirror of his Being with her.

## Awareness and its Implications for Practice

Clients' awareness goes beyond that which we call conscious awareness, because all awareness is embodied. Sometimes our bodies are wiser than our conscious minds. Those things which are put out of conscious or focused awareness are present within the psychophysical matrix of the self.

Because the therapist who strives to understand all of awareness as a mirror of Being accesses at some level this embodied information, then there arises a curious dilemma about power. Every person-centred therapist needs to wrestle with this as a dilemma. If the dilemma is avoided, so is the power issue.

Let us agree that as far as possible the therapist aims to equalize the power balance within the therapeutic relationship. Paradoxically, this is a very powerful position to be in. In much work, the therapist does have at first a privileged understanding of power dynamics. The client who starts on an equal footing here is rare. The therapist is more powerful both because of her expertise in the therapeutic relationship and because she is more congruent than the client (Rogers, 1957a, conditions two and three). In addition to this inherent problem with power, the therapist strives to understand the client's awareness, some of which is out of the client's consciousness. This level of understanding is at the heart of depth reflection as put forward by Thorne and Mearns' four-point empathy scale (Mearns and Thorne, 1999, pp. 44–8).

The therapist's dilemma is this. If the knowledge of what is going on within the client's processing is never actively offered to the client's reflexive awareness then, although this may seem to be more classically and non-directively person-centred, it maintains a privileged position for the therapist. I do not offer this argument lightly. It is not clear-cut. It is not 'clever'. There are of course counter-arguments. Rather it is an invitation to wrestle with the subtleties of the power dynamic of awareness.

In Chapter 11, I will suggest that the existential element of person-centred therapy is at its most potent only when the client has developed and can hold a knowledge of her own process – see there the case study of Heather. The therapists reflexive awareness of the client's embodied awarenesses is a double-edged sword. Person-Centred therapists must wield it with care. (The sword image is not a natural one for person-centred work.) The literalist cannot avoid the dilemma, nor the experientialist afford to be cavalier about it.

In the next chapter the phenomenological perspective moves our attention from the client's process to that of the therapist. The philosophical commitment to phenomenology is seen as leading to a freeing of the therapist's way of being.

## Further Reading

Harris, J.B. (2003) *Gestalt: A New Idiosyncratic Introduction*. Manchester, Gestalt Centre (3rd edition).

An outstanding small book which gives in an accessible and experiential form a very good understanding of Gestalt therapy.

Perls, F.S. (1992) *Gestalt Therapy Verbatim*. Gouldsboro, ME, Gestalt Journal Press.

A lively and important insight into how Fritz Perls used to do therapy. Good to know rather than to imitate.

Perls, F.S., R.F. Hefferline and P. Goodman (1973) *Gestalt Therapy: Excitement and Growth in the Human Personality*. Harmondsworth, Penguin.

Still the definitive work on Gestalt therapy. Authoritative but a tough read.

Sills, C., S. Fish and P. Lapworth (1995) *Gestalt Counselling*. Bicester, Winslow Press.

A fulsome book which brings it all together, experience and theory. Perhaps the one of them all to own.

Stephens, J.O. (1989) *Awareness*. London, Eden Grove.

A book rich in experiments in personal awareness. Gestalt theory in practice.

# 8

# Freeing the Therapist: A Phenomenological Reading of Carl Rogers

So far, the focus has been on the client relationship as it is informed by an increased awareness of phenomenological principles. The client's frame of reference is not just a technical question of accurate empathy, but is at the heart of understanding how we know about others at all. The client's process is one aspect of the phenomena which compose her frame of reference. Thus it is necessary to address the client's process to be open to the whole of her frame of reference. The contents of the client's frame of reference is both reflexive and spontaneous, both in and out of her focused awareness. The therapist has an unavoidable choice on any occasion about whether to engage process rather than content as the primary focus of empathy. This is a difficult choice, but a creative one. Rather than see the choice as directive, it can be worked with as another route to trusting the client's actualizing tendency. It is implicit in Rogers (1957c) that the client's experience of her own process both spontaneously and reflexively is to be trusted as one aspect of the expression of her tendency to self-actualize.

So far, the focus has been on the therapist's relationship with the client. In this and the next chapter, the concern will be the therapist's relationship with herself. I will argue that a phenomenological reading of Carl Rogers leads to a therapist self-identity which is permissive of the adventure of person-centred process work.

In arguing that the writings of Carl Rogers must be read phenomenologically, we move away from a conventional educational model, an oppressive one, in which the contents of what is read constitute an external authority to which I must conform. Rather, the act of reading produces a synthesis of therapist-with-Carl Rogers.

This in turn frees us to explore and, above all, to become ourselves in the acts and relationships of therapy. In engaging with therapeutic theory at a deeply phenomenological level, the therapist is released to construct responsibly a practice that is truly personal.

I begin with a return to the nature of phenomenological awareness:

---

**Personal Focus 8.1    An act of phenomenological awareness**

I pick up my late mother's engagement ring, with its solitaire diamond. I know in my head that it is brilliant-cut – a technical terms meaning that it is cut with 64 faces to give the best effect. As I look at it I can make the mistake that I see the diamond itself. I do not. I see only part, but even what I do see, I see only through my own eyes, my own sense-perceptions. The more I meditate on this, the more I come to know that the diamond-in-itself is remote, inaccessible to me. Beyond this is the fact that I have a whole range of seeings of the diamond which compose Richard-with-the-diamond. I see it in its claw-settings. I can count the faces I see, and then turn it to count more. I can see its yellow fire. I can feel its hardness, and perhaps even see that hardness in the fineness of its cut. I can look through its surface for its inner colour and its one interior blemish. Yet I see beyond this; for above all, it is my late mother's. It is what Jack gave to Kath in 1949. It embodies their love, and mine for them. When my wife wears it, there is a flow across the generations. It will, I hope, continue to belong to my children when I am dead. I see a living symbol built on my memory and deep feeling.

---

## Experiencing Looking

Phenomenology teaches us that there are no convincing boundaries between the 'world-out-there' and the world that we construct. Our one certainty is that we cannot know where the objective and subjective contact each other. They intertwine. The diamond is real; it is not just an aspect of the onlooker. Yet it is beyond the grasp of the onlooker. The real diamond, though, is also more impoverished than the object of the phenomenological field – the diamond-as-I-see-it. For my version of the diamond 'contains' not just a limited knowledge of the real diamond, but also the whole set of thoughts and feelings which I have for it, as well as the personal and social constructs that are contingent upon it. By way of example, the diamond not only contains my love for my parents, a personal construct, but also the fact that I am an only child living in a society in which both property and identity are passed down the generations.

In short, it is not possible for me to encounter the diamond without my constructing a complex object which I call Richard-with-the-diamond. There are parts of this construct which are incorrigibly my own, such as my feelings for my mother. There are other parts which are allied to this but which are factually present; the diamond belongs to me and is not a fake. These are linked by my spontaneous and reflexive acts of experiencing.

As with the diamond, so with the work of Carl Rogers. When I am properly aware of phenomenological reading, I know that I am released into, and cannot escape, the creation of Richard-with-Carl Rogers. In exploring this act of reading, I hope to contact my freedom and need to be myself as a therapist.

## Phenomenological Reading

When I read a text with phenomenological awareness, I am not so much concerned about what the text 'says' – true or false. Rather I am interested in, and aware of, how that text impacts upon me. The key concept here is not so much 'known truth' as 'lived truth'. Meaning comes to exist within a dialogue between the text and the reader, with all of her life-experience. Rogers always invites his readers to take his theory and his experiencing as a hypothesis to use in their own lives. Therefore, a phenomenological reading of Rogers is a risk, and a risk that requires a degree of maturity in the therapist, a sense of her own growing competence. When I read phenomenologically, I can no longer ask, what does Rogers teach me? Rather, I must ask, how, when I meet Rogers, am I changed? In reading in this spirit, I do not become 'Rogerian'. I become more myself as a thinking, feeling, researching, experimenting, person-centred therapist. While it is not widely discussed, this change from an external to an internal locus of creativity-as-therapist is a vital aspect of therapist education, and of the growth of the reflective practitioner.

This process of reading can be opened up in terms of the contrast between spontaneity and reflexivity, and in this to-ing and fro-ing. I parallel client process. When I read Rogers with phenomenological awareness, I attempt to move from reflexivity, what do I think his argument is? To spontaneity, how am I changed by him? And thence back to reflexivity, how do I now act as a therapist? (This resembles the experiential learning model of Kolb, 1984. See Chapter 1.)

---

**Personal Focus 8.2    Reflexive and spontaneous awareness**

Humans are reflexive because we are aware – and we are aware that we are aware. I know I am conscious. I can grasp the future.

I know I will die. I can know that I cause things to happen. Sometimes I think too hard for my own good. All of these elements of reflexivity are at the heart of the humanistic vision. Humans are spontaneous because they can live in immediate touch with their organismic potential, because they are more than mere intellect, because they can escape from their reflexivity, because body and mind are a single system, because thoughts are felt and emotions known. To be healthy is to hold a balance as well as a tension between these two components of being. I need to be reflexive, aware at a high level; I need to be spontaneous, to feel my own free flow of experiencing without seeing it only from the balcony of the conscious mind. Rogers' various descriptions of healthy process seem to me to do admirable justice to our need to find an authentic way of living with this tension between reflexivity and spontaneity.

With this in mind, contact a piece of learning, such as riding a bicycle or learning to drive.

- What part of your learning was reflexive in the first instance? What purpose did that serve?
- What part of your learning was spontaneous and at the edge of awareness in the first instance? What purpose did that serve?
- When did you move from one mode to the other? What is your sense of the purpose of this movement?

Just as I experience Rogers through what he has written, and the taped work of him I have seen – I do not 'understand', for he is closer to me than that – this Rogers-experience becomes an element in my experience of myself, my life-values, my work, my clients and so forth. As I experience Rogers-in-my-context, then some of what he talks about stands out for me. In the light of living and counselling, I notice themes, arguments, observations which matter to me. This act of noticing incorporates the textures and structures of my experiencing. It is in no way value-free or objective. Reading Rogers subjectively is congruent with the whole heritage of humanistic therapy and psychology. As Carol Becker (1992, p. 8) points out, the aim of awareness is to be 'efficient and effective participants in life'. As I truly engage with Rogers, I interact with him to become a better therapist (Worsley, 1997).

My plea to read Rogers in the light of the phenomenological principle is neither a licence to make of him something detached from objective reality nor a deconstruction of him into total relativization. Edmund Husserl was quite clear that our experiencing is of real objects in a real and above all interpersonal world:

> I experience the world (including others) and, according to its experiential sense, not as (so to speak) my *private* synthetic formation but as other than mine alone, as an *intersubjective* world, actually there for everyone, accessible in respect of its Objects to everyone.
>
> (1977, p. 91)

My reading of Rogers only exists in the context of the scholarly and therapeutic communities to which reader and author belong and are joined. I must be a responsible reader – and therapist. Yet the experience is still subjective, deeply personal and formative. When I choose to read and write about Rogers in conscious awareness of the phenomenological method, this is one variety of the tension between reflexivity and spontaneity. I must think hard about how I think in order that I can spontaneously engage with Rogers-as-he-is-to-me. This version of Rogers is governed by what interests me.

## Two Ways of Looking at Rogers

What difference does a phenomenological reading of Rogers make?

Phenomenological reading is not about some sloppy subjectivism. It is based on a hard-headed theory of knowledge. If I think I can grasp the thing-in-itself, I am mistaken. I can only know the thing-as-it-is-to-me. Yet this gives a richer and more mature knowledge. I let go of the illusion that I see the diamond. I have only my-seeing-the-diamond. In the same way, a mature reading of Rogers is to move from the illusion that an objective sets of facts constitutes Rogers' theory, towards the experience of feeling and knowing the impact that his work makes upon me. I am freed to respond.

Rogers the empiricist invites us to take his experiences and what he calls low-level theory, and to use them as a hypothesis for our living. I want to illustrate this way of reading by contrasting it with the account of Rogers' theory in Thorne (1992). This is not a criticism of a really useful book, but rather points to the limitations of all introductory texts.

In chapter two, Thorne offers a coherent account of Rogers' theory. I believe we are invited to read it as a brief rendition of what we are to *understand* if we are to enter into a therapeutically effective relationship with the client. The chapter offers eight sections, each of which can be reduced to a proposition, so that these string together to form a coherent argument. The first five might read:

---

### Box 8.1 Five themes from Thorne (1992)

Subjective experience is central to being a person, and as such is trustworthy because we behave in accordance with our perceptions of the world as we see it.

Each person is governed by an 'actualizing tendency' which leads them naturally to strive to fulfil their own potential. However, the way each of us believes ourselves to be – our self-concept – is distorted, and as such inhibits our actualizing tendency. In other words, there is an incongruence internally between the actualizing tendency and aspects of the self-concept.

This incongruence or distortion springs from the conditions of worth imposed on us throughout life, but in particular in early childhood. We introject the message: You will only be loved/accepted IF....

This distortion means that we tend to evaluate ourselves, our actions and others in terms of these introjects, which come to make up the structure of our self-concept: I am bad when I tell a truth that will hurt Mummy. An external locus of evaluation signals an incongruence between our organismic need and how we act. As the locus of evaluation is internalized, congruence both within the self and with others and the world increases.

In therapy and in life the actualizing tendency leads us towards a process of being 'fully functioning'. This is a process or direction and not a state or goal, and as such will differ from person to person.

---

Brian Thorne writes,

The first and most striking characteristic of the 'fully functioning person' as Rogers describes him or her is an increasing openness to experience. Such individuals are able to listen to themselves and to others and to allow themselves to experience what is happening without feeling threatened. Secondly, they have the ability to live fully in the present and to be attentive to each moment as it is lived.

(Thorne, 1992, p. 34)

There then follow three points concerning the core conditions and their place within the therapeutic relationship. However, I want to draw attention to the overall quality of the statement of the argument, the summary of Rogers' system of thought, and then contrast it with the quotation in the preceding paragraph.

The five propositions above form a relatively coherent argument, which students in person-centred counselling need to come to understand. The intellectual grasp of these enables the student to see why the implementation of the core conditions is important, and, through a grasp of the nature of incongruence, to see how a client's material may relate to their desire to change. As the grasp becomes more sophisticated and more rooted in experience of client work, the counsellor is increasingly able to empathize, to accept and to be appropriately congruent, while formulating within themselves a more and more tuned-in version of the client's world. This is good initial learning. But it is learning only to apply and use an intellectual construct. Rogerian theory remains 'truth'. Insight is another matter.

Let us return to the few sentences of Brian Thorne's, quoted above: 'The client becomes more fully functioning when she becomes more open to experience, and can live more fully in the present.' It is not obvious from the stated theory why these two phenomena should signal fuller function. The reason, of course, is that Rogers did not *deduce* them from theory. He arrived at them *inductively, empirically,* by reflecting openly on the experience of clients who had found therapy beneficial. This is his phenomenological method.

Thus to read Rogers phenomenologically is to trust to my own maturity and grounding in person-centredness so as to 'let go' of theory and explore my own experience in the light of my reading. The 'truth' of Rogers transforms into the insight of Richard-reading-Rogers. I am freed to discover how I might address the client's process and my own while aspiring to remain true to Sanders' (2000) primary and secondary principles (Boxes 2.1 and 2.2). My freedom allows me to note where I fall short of the primary set and enter clearly into therapeutic error, and where I fall short of the secondary set and thus choose either to correct my practice or to redefine my position.

With this freedom appreciated, one particular quality of person-centred theory points to the need to engage client process. This quality I call the person-centred theory paradox.

## The Person-Centred Theory Paradox and Openness to the Client's Process

Not long after completing his milestone book, *Client-Centered Therapy,* Rogers, together with his co-researcher Dymond, wrote,

> One of the major theoretical hypotheses of client-centered therapy is that during therapy the concept of the self is revised to assimilate basic experiences which had previously been denied to awareness as threatening.
>
> (Rogers and Dymond, 1954, p. 13)

According to Rogers (1957a), the six conditions of therapy are both necessary and sufficient for the change in self-concept to occur. The six conditions are conditions of relating, and as such do not map directly to any content of that relationship (Tudor, 2000). Thus the paradox of person-centred therapy is that the therapy itself need not overtly address the issues that are at the root of the dysfunctional self-concept. Rogers nowhere claims that a conscious addressing of the conditions of worth or of the locus of evaluation of the client is necessary for significant psychological change to occur.

This fact is not at all surprising when we reflect that those aspects of our personality structures which are healthy stem from early life-experiences of the core conditions in such a way as to keep us in touch with our organismic valuing process. We do not necessarily address issues of function and dysfunction at the conscious level during the natural processes of growth and maturation. This fact and my experiences with some of my clients lead me to suppose that the paradox of person-centred therapy embodies an important truth. The key changes to the client *can* all take place outside of, or perhaps at the edge of, the client's awareness. I want to make an important distinction here, however. Almost all clients will be aware of change at least at the level of Gendlin's felt-sense. My claim here is that this awareness will not necessarily enter into the fullness of their thinking.

Person-Centred therapy may be unique in that the key issues for the client can all be sufficiently addressed without these entering the conscious system. This paradox is another version of the reflexivity-spontaneity continuum.

When the client experiences change as a direct and immediate result of the therapeutic relationship, there is a spontaneous growth in the depth and flow of feelings and in a homogenous, mind–body awareness (Gendlin, 1981). Such clients will sometimes be naïvely unaware of the nature of the therapeutic process and will speak of feeling stronger and relieved by a chance to talk. By contrast, some clients experience a close and difficult confrontation with their conditions of worth, the sources of these, their operationalization within their self-evaluating processes, and the links between their emotions and their thinking and belief systems. People are different; they process differently. Some people seem to experience the corrective processes engendered within the therapeutic relationship as spontaneous, and at the edge of their awareness; others fight through these processes in a highly reflexive fashion. Each, it would seem to me, is valid. More than that, any individual is likely to process somewhere on a continuum between spontaneity and reflexivity, and to move along parts of this continuum in a pendulum-like fashion.

It might be that some clients need or invite process work, while others do not. The client will alert me to the possibility of person-centred process work. I want to trust my client's unconscious knowledge of her ability and need to engage at this level. Process work is not a contradiction of the necessity and sufficiency of the core conditions, but an implementation of those conditions, just to the extent that process work is congruent with, and motivated by, the client's actualizing tendency and that the therapist can hear it as such.

## Conceptualizing and Operationalizing

I have put forward a reading of Carl Rogers which first suggests that the subjective experience of operationalizing what I know of Rogers is far more powerful than academic debate normally allows. I meet my clients with an experiential integration of Richard-and-Carl Rogers. I have argued elsewhere that this is inevitable (Worsley, 1997). The question of therapist behaviour is inescapable. I reject the implication of some purists that process work is an abandonment of the necessity and sufficiency of the core conditions, and that process work is a plunge into instrumentalism – tools-instead-of-relating.

Therapists both conceptualize and operationalize. We have a choice. I may know X but consciously choose not to act upon it; I may know Y and not be conscious of whether or not this affects my actions; I may know Z and decide to act upon it.

At a practical level, this is an important distinction. I take it as an axiom of my own practice, and of the use of supervision in particular, that while I may be at the spontaneous end of our continuum when with my client, I need to be reflexive when giving an account of what I do and how I am. Given the choice, it is more responsible to act consciously than unconsciously.

I profoundly doubt that a therapist is wholly unaffected by a deeper knowledge of client process. It is ethically important to know and decide how this knowledge is operationalized. We have less choice than we might imagine about whether or not we operationalize knowledge. Therefore the question is inescapable as to how we as therapists operationalize our knowledge of client process.

The core conditions are not actions or deeds. They are qualities of relating. They subsist in actions. For instance, in skills training, empathy might be seen to subsist in paraphrasing or in reflecting feeling. Rogers was of course quite right that reflecting feeling is not the same as empathy, and that skills alone do not make a therapist person-centred (Rogers, 1986b). Skills alone can lead to a portrayal of the core conditions, but genuineness in relating requires a movement forward of considerable proportion (Mearns, 1997, pp. 27–8). Therefore, no particular action can be said in and of itself to breach the necessity and sufficiency or the core conditions unless it can be shown to fail to embody the core conditions. Process work is potentially an expression of the core conditions of therapy.

I contrast this stance with one condemned – rightly I believe – by Jerold Bozarth (1998). He describes five typical distortions of person-centred therapy. The third is that the therapist is an expert on the client's process, with the result that:

> [t]he therapist now knows where the client should go, and knows the natural idiosyncratic process of that particular client, and (depending on the therapist's bent to be an expert) is now in a theoretical position to direct the client through the 'proper and right' process.
>
> (Bozarth, 1998, p. 24)

If it is the case that to be an expert (and that is a loaded word) on process is to know where the client ought to go, then that is directive in the sense that it withdraws trust and autonomy from the client's own actualizing tendency, and hence is contrary to person-centred practice.

However, it is *not* clear that process expertise has these consequences at all. If I am an 'expert' on process, first I can recognize process and then make responsible decisions on how I can and cannot respond to it. In just the same way, the person-centred therapist is an 'expert' on relating because she is 'congruent or integrated in the relationship' – one of Rogers' six conditions of therapy (Rogers, 1957a, p. 96). This does not mean that she directs the client in relating. She offers an open relationship with appropriate expertise. Expertise in the person-centred sense is at the heart of therapy, and includes a full trusting of the client's actualizing tendency.

A phenomenological reading of the texts of Carl Rogers can move the therapist towards an internal locus of therapeutic judgement. She is freed from the travails of orthodoxy to a more reflective stance, and above all she is liberated into a practice which is truly personal. To use Rogers' own word, it is idiosyncratic (Rogers, 1978, pp. 205–6).

---

**Personal Focus 8.3   Freeing up my identity as a therapist**

It is clear that no other person can determine how we practise at the level of our own identity. Unless we own and work critically with our therapeutic identity, we will continue to export our locus of evaluation as therapists, and project it onto the system or approach to which we adhere. Ironic!

I address the readers presuming that they are practising therapists. In cases where this is not true, this process of working with identity may well still be of use.

I offer a number of statements designed in differing degrees to be contentious. How do you respond? What awareness comes for you about the roots of your therapeutic identity?

- I am person-centred because I have faith in it as a belief-system.
- I am person-centred because that reflects my personal journey in therapy, and may well correspond to my personality-type.
- My position within the person-centred movement has remained more or less constant over time.
- People who shift position really haven't got the underlying principles sorted out.
- Eclecticism is the main threat to our identity as a movement.
- I read Rogers' texts to find out what it is to be truly person-centred.
- I am still discovering what it is to be person-centred.
- Some practitioners are open and accepting of all, except for other person-centred practitioners with whom they disagree.
- I express all of me as a person in meeting my clients.
- My own practice reflects who I want to be. It's fine to be called idiosyncratic.

I know what frees me to be myself as a therapist.

In this chapter, phenomenological reading has brought us back to themes which have already occurred in the book. In the following chapters, a new theme will emerge: phenomenology leads on to the existential basis of counselling.

## Further Reading

Barrett-Lennard, G.T. (1998) *Carl Rogers' Helping System: Journey and Substance.* London, Sage. Chapter 15.

In a single chapter, Goff Barrett-Lennard gets to the heart of training as personal growth and hence as freedom to be. It sits well within this long and authoritative history of the thought of the person-centred movement.

Hobson, R.F. (1985) *Forms of Feeling: The Heart of Psychotherapy.* London, Tavistock.

Hobson looks at therapy from a Jungian training, but offers an account of his Conversational Model which cuts across the modalities of therapy, and is highly compatible with person-centred thought. It is perhaps the most inspiring and intensely focused account I know of the role of the therapist as partner in encounter. In this work, it is crucial to be free to be oneself.

Shlien, J.M. (2003) 'To Feel Alive: A Thought on Motivation'. In P. Sanders (ed.) *To Lead an Honorable Life: Invitations to Think about Client-Centered Therapy and the Person-Centered Approach*. Ross-on-Wye, PCCS Books. Chapter 1.

A crisp and novel statement of what it might mean to be free to express oneself as a person.

Tudor, K. and Worrall, M. (eds.) (2004) *Freedom to Practice: Person-Centred Approaches to Supervision*. Ross-on-Wye, PCCS Books.

While this book is overtly about supervision, it is therefore about the whole of therapeutic practice. I simply record that for me it does what it aims to, as stated in its introduction (p. 6): it seeks to encourage the reader to 'to reflect, and to think and to question; to roam, trespass and transgress; to be curious, critical and creative'.

# Part III
## Existential Perspectives

# 9

# Relating and Existing: Martin Buber's I–Thou Construct for Person-Centred Therapy

This chapter is about the idea of relating, particularly as seen through the eyes of Martin Buber. Martin Buber is perhaps the most important Jewish theologian of the twentieth century, but he is also a significant secular philosopher who has contributed much to our understanding of relating. For those who follow in the footsteps of Carl Rogers, the importance of the therapeutic relationship is evident. Here I attempt to understand it in the light of Buber's thinking. Buber's ideas about relating are an indispensable bridge to existential awareness.

Relating is one key aspect of what it is to exist as human beings. Person-centred therapy depends heavily on existential thinking as well as upon the phenomenological thinking that we have already explored. In Kirschenbaum and Henderson (1990b) we have a record of Rogers' dialogues with seven of the age's key thinkers. Of these, three are major figures in existentialist philosophy and theology – Paul Tillich, Martin Buber and Rollo May – while even Reinhold Niebuhr, a theological colleague of Tillich's, falls approximately within this school of thinking. This chapter and the next aim to open up the practical significance of thinking existentially as well as phenomenologically.

The aims of this chapter are essentially practical: how, in the light of Buber's thinking, can we understand the case of Hannah, the office bully? However, in order to see the point of Buber's work, we will need some map of the road that leads from phenomenology to existentialism. Therefore, the practical section is preceded by a brief examination of two questions: Why think existentially? What is existentialism? My teaching colleagues and I are increasingly convinced that in counsellor education a basic grasp of the underlying philosophy is crucial in keeping therapists in touch with the undergirding principles of their practice. It is tough-going, but worth it.

# From Phenomenology to Existentialism

So far we have looked at phenomenology as a broadly useful theory of knowing, which confirms the commitment of person-centred therapy to work largely within the client's frame of reference, and to renounce the possibility of counsellor expertise upon the client's world. The therapist is encouraged in this way to be self-aware in bracketing off pre-judgements of the client's world, and to have a keen appreciation of the very different ways in which human beings construct their world views, both as individuals and as members of social groups and communities.

Behind this workaday thinking lies a number of unaddressed, technical questions. A major one must concern us now. For Husserl, the act of bracketing out, of discarding all presuppositions, is not just a matter of good method. It stems from his conclusion that all consciousness is 'intentional', that is to say, is consciousness of something. This in turn leads him to conclude that there must be something which is conscious that is still there when it is empty of all content. He calls it the transcendental ego. Husserl has been criticized for holding to an idea of the self which is difficult because it reduces all other selves to mere sense impressions. Yet as with Buber himself, we need a view of reality which does justice to the existence of others like us: 'A conscious self always entails a sense of others' (Crossley, 1996, p. 9). This means that I assemble my own identity only in a social context. I have no self-identity if it is not for my being part of a group, a tribe, a community, a society. To cut a long story short, we exist because we exist with others who were there from our beginning.

Existentialism takes very seriously this sense of the word 'exist'. In this specialist sense, only human beings exist, and existence is a property of humanity in general. To exist is to stand out over against the rest of the universe, to be different. That difference is in our ability to be conscious of the self, and to be conscious of the act of being conscious of the self. You will recognize this as Rennie's term 'reflexivity', which is contrasted in previous chapters with spontaneity. For some existentialists, in particular Sartre, we stand out by virtue of what we do in the concrete world. This process can be approximately equated with 'taking responsibility for ourselves'.

Existentialism or rather existential phenomenology differs from Husserl's version of phenomenology because it points to concrete reality and to our standing out as humans in the universe with others. Only when we take a broadly existentialist stance can we see the self as at heart relational.

To see the self as relational is a prerequisite of Rogers' own thought, for the necessity and sufficiency of the therapeutic conditions both imply and require a view of humanity as constituted in relationship with others. Without others' regard and empathy, we do not come to exist.

I am aware that in the last six paragraphs, I have compacted a very substantial argument into a small space. The core of it is that we need existential thinking to see why people only come into being in relationship. This rather abstract thought will become more rooted and imaginable as this and the next chapter proceed.

## What is Existentialism?

> Philosophy is a product of the humanity of each philosopher, and each philosopher is a man of flesh and bone who addresses himself to other men of flesh and bone like himself. And, let him do what he will, he philosophizes not with the reason only, but with the will, with the feelings, with the flesh and the bones, with the whole soul and with the whole body.
>
> (Unamuno, 1954, p. 28, cited in Macquarrie, 1972/1991, p. 15)

The person-centred therapist has much in common with the words, above, of Miguel de Unamuno. Existentialism is above all a philosophy of the human. It faces in depth what it is to be human. I suggest that the therapist must also be wrestling with this question. In order to accompany another human being on her journey towards wholeness, we must have some inkling of what the humanity is for which we quest.

For the existentialist, being human is rooted in the nature of existence. Jean-Paul Sartre puts it thus:

> We mean that man (*sic*) first of all exists, encounters himself, surges up in the world – and defines himself afterwards. If man, as the existentialist sees him, is not definable, it is because to begin with he is nothing. He will not be anything until later, and then he will be what he makes of himself.
>
> (Sartre, *L'existentialisme est un humanisme*, cited in Kaufman, 1956, p. 289)

We 'surge up in the world' because there is no core, intellectual self in the way that Descartes had envisaged. We surge up by our recognizing our responsibility to live authentically (whatever that might turn out to mean). We are alive in a world in which there are no rules and values handed down from on high, but rather in which we have to take responsibility for ourselves.

It would be wrong to think that these words have only one meaning. It is one of the challenges of existentialist thinking that it is so diverse. None of the great tomes on the subject actually contains the word 'existentialism' (Cooper,

1990, p. 1). Most existentialists would rather not be called so. There is much confusion as to the meaning of the word. Some thinkers like Camus probably do not warrant the term 'existentialist', and yet have been deeply influential (Cooper, 1990, pp. 11–19). Existentialism rejects rules handed down from on high and yet many existentialists are believers in God. In spite of all this diversity, the theme of responsibility is a thread to lead us through much of this jungle of thought.

This radical responsibility for the self comes in many guises. Sartre sees it as the radical fidelity to our unfettered freedom. If God were to exist, he argues, that would compromise freedom. Kierkegaard, while seeing that all truths must relate to our own existential emergence, and therefore cannot be absolute, can place this relativity of truth in the context of a firm and personal faith in God. The God of Kierkegaard invites us to step beyond the ethical, the rule-bound, into what Kierkegaard calls the absurd in order to be in a faithful relationship (Gardiner, 1996, pp. 71–9).

For the German philosopher of Being, Martin Heidegger, the key category is thrownness. According to Heidegger, thrownness is the quality of being alive in our world such that we had no choice about the matter. We exist. We can choose the mode of our existence but not the fact of our existence. (Even death and suicide are aspects of our thrownness.) From this thrownness comes existential anxiety, that sense of being ill-at-ease in life. Heidegger notes that people try to evade this anxiety at their thrownness by objectifying the world (Polt, 1999, p. 67).

The therapist can recognize what he means here in the language that is associated with conditions of worth. 'We really cannot displease our mothers, can we?' In so saying, we express not just our conditions of worth but an attempt at a universal rule. In making this pseudo-rule, that no mother can be displeased, we seek to abnegate our personal responsibility. Personal responsibility is the decision that, having recognized our conditions of worth, we will continue to live by them or overthrow them. We project this responsibility out away from ourselves so that it becomes a sort of absolute, social rule of behaviour. If all behaviour were socially governed and indisputable like this, there would be certitude. There is not. Our thrownness manifests itself in our anxiety at the lack of certitude that comes from our having no choice but to make choices, even if by default.

The challenge then is to live authentically. (What a counsellor might mean by this will be the subject of the next chapter.) For Heidegger, this authenticity subsists in concern. Concern is a difficult word. It includes taking care and being careful, heedfulness, caring for others, giving proper attention to the self. Concern is both abstract and is to be lived out in the practical and concrete aspects of life. It is above all about the way that we relate to our living, to the very project of being alive.

This links to the more practical existential matters dealt with in therapy. Yalom (1980; 1989) focuses especially upon death and anxiety, freedom, isolation and meaninglessness. Cohn (1997) adds to this: anxiety and guilt, sexuality, withdrawal and authentic living. Paul Tillich (1952) provides a particularly stimulating account of the philosophical bases of anxiety, based on three pairs of concepts: fate and death; emptiness and meaninglessness; guilt and condemnation. He suggests that the first member of each pair is an everyday 'cover' for the second member. This second member is the more absolute existential crisis.

Buber asks us to consider in depth the ways in which we live in radical relatedness with each other. We shall explore the case of Hannah as a way into understanding how Buber can help us empathize in depth with our clients.

### Case 9.1 Hannah

Hannah was referred to me by the personnel department of the agency for which she works. The referral mentioned unsatisfactory work performance linked to her problematic use of alcohol. She was a single woman in her mid-forties.

Hannah was in fact the manager of a fairly large section of her agency. In the previous two-and-a-half years, she had experienced a very high turnover of staff under her. Her immediate senior saw it as a problem of her drinking leading to an attitude that was both demanding and aggressive. She set her staff notoriously high standards and, when they failed to match them, she would respond punitively, and at times with ill-concealed rage. Her junior colleagues therefore both feared and despised her.

When I first met Hannah, I was struck by her smart, polished appearance, lacking any soft edge to it. She seemed to be very much the business-person, but the veneer displayed no flexibility. I have come over the years to have some sense early on as to whether a self-presentation is defensive or not. My first impression of Hannah was that she needed to be seen as sharp, efficient, glossy. I wondered what she feared others might discover beneath this surface. After a few minutes of being in her company, I began to recognize that I was responding to her 'body-armour'. She held her musculature tense, postured. It seemed that it would not be possible for her to be in my company and be relaxed. As I watched her, I noticed that the tension seemed to function in a very different way from those who present with stress or panic. With the latter, tension seems like a burden, exhausting. I want to work my own muscles to help them to relax. Their tension is like steel bands holding them in. For Hannah, the tension seemed so much more part of her, just one more aspect of her veneer. I felt it in her caution, her wariness. She held herself eternally vigilant. I have heard the saying that eternal vigilance is the cost of freedom. I wondered what was the pay-off for Hannah's aggressive-defensive patrolling of the boundaries of her own body.

As I worked to get to know Hannah in the early days of our relationship – and it felt like hard work – I came to recognize that her bullying was part of a complex defensive structure. She had come to despise her employees much as they despised her. She knew how they felt. She hated them at times, but more often she hated herself. She worked for a number of weeks with the theme of control. Bullying was a 'safe' way of controlling the environment for which she was responsible. As I reflected her own fear in doing this, I felt first of all her resistance to the idea that she had emotional reasons to bully. Could I not just teach her to be a better manager? Yet, in persisting, I noticed a softening in her, as if she were questioning whether to trust me enough to confess that she was hurting.

Beneath the controlling behaviour Hannah feared that she was out of control. She had, she told me eventually, a drink problem. (She had not seen an alcohol worker. It was not yet clear to me that this would be at all necessary.) Hannah drank whisky and gin – about 40 units a week. She had a marked pattern of consumption. She would be able to spend an evening or a weekend in her flat without drinking at all. She even joked that her preferred addiction when alone was Chinese food! Her consumption had a binge-like quality to it. Occasionally she would drink early in the day to cover up 'her nerves', and then, racked with guilt, would abstain rigidly. I remember feeling that the rigidity of her withdrawal and self-disgust echoed her way of relating to her colleagues. Perhaps she bullied herself too. Her main consumption was with friends or by herself at her golf-club. The bar attendant there had got quite used to calling her a taxi when she became helpless. She had developed quite a social reputation as a hard drinker. Her friends often showed concern, but she kept them well at bay.

It was week seven of our work before Hannah began to tell me of her parents. Again she felt guilt. They had given her in many ways an ideal childhood, at least in material terms. Her father, however, was constantly absent. He worked in the leisure industry in a senior post that took him abroad constantly. When he did come home, he never seemed present to her. He was continually escaping Hannah's mother, whose behaviour was persistently anxious, demanding of attention and at times insecure and dependent. She was constantly jealous of her husband's freedom, and suspected him of being unfaithful to her. The emotional environment of Hannah's rearing was cold, with-holding and fearful. It was not difficult to see that what Hannah had experienced she readily reproduced in her own personal relating. The surface appearances had come to predominate. Good manners were paramount; concern had little place.

## Deeper Empathy

I am by now quite clear in my own mind that I need to conceptualize the client in a number of ways in order to gain a deeper appreciation of her position. Constructs, ways of thinking about the client, can never be more than intelligent guesses as to how it is for the client. The therapist needs to check out this understanding with the client. Constructs, ideas about the client's world, pictures of how life is for her open up possibilities for empathy, for the questioning of my understanding the richness and detail of the client's experiencing.

If I can come to understand something of Hannah's bullying, I will develop a greater sense of the emotions which underlie the behaviour, emotions against which she needs to defend. I can never know that I am right, nor is it my task to break down anyone's defences. I need mine! I presume others do too. Yet, I can empathize with the fear which the behaviour betrays. I will do so carefully, tentatively, and without any sense that this is what the client 'ought' to feel.

Let us return to the main claim of the existential perspective, that we stand out from the universe by virtue of our authenticity and our relatedness, and our embeddedness in the concrete world. Buber's concept of the I–Thou over against the I–It offers us a category by which to understand the structure of Hannah's world. What are the I–Thou relationships and what are the I–It relationships? When I can understand something of how Hannah exists (in that technical sense of the word), I have a deeper empathy with her. Only when I can have empathy can I risk challenging her at the level of her authenticity.

## A View of Hannah – Martin Buber

Buber is both an existentialist philosopher and a Jewish theologian. His key ideas, which have contributed greatly to our understanding of what it is to be human, are not difficult, but the reading of his work – even his slim volume *I and Thou* – is very demanding. In this brief space, I will pay attention only to a small number of his key ideas.

René Descartes' aphorism *cogito ergo sum* – I think therefore I am – has governed much philosophy since the Enlightenment. Humans are seen as being essentially individuals who are defined by the act of thinking, of cognition. Buber rejects the notion that we are distilled centres of intellect. He believes that we are essentially relational.

For Buber, this relational character of humanity is derived from our primary relationship with God. It is, however, not necessary to take on board the theological part of Buber's argument to benefit from his anthropology (Crossley, 1996, pp. 10–11). Buber's thinking approximates to that of Melanie Klein and the object relations school, the basic presupposition of which is that we are born with a drive to relate. Buber takes this analysis of our primary need to relate a step beyond the psychodynamic description. He is the more radical, for he sees not a Single that needs to relate, but believes humanity is essentially dyadic. We subsist first and foremost in the I–Thou. Relating is more basic, more fundamental than the unitary individual.

Buber argues that we should not think of ourselves as 'I':

> To man (*sic*) the world is twofold, in accordance with his twofold attitude.
> The attitude of man is twofold, in accordance with the twofold nature of the primary words which he speaks.
> The primary words are not isolated words, but combined words.
> The one primary word is the combination *I–Thou*,
> The other primary word is the combination *I–It* . . . .
> Primary words do not signify things, but they intimate relations.
> Primary words do not describe something that might exist independently of them, but being spoken they bring about existence.
>
> (Buber, 1958, p. 15)

This famous opening to *I and Thou* is deceptively simple. In it, Buber makes three profoundly important observations. The first is that how humans see the world is based upon a common-sense notion that we treat the world habitually in two different ways. Some aspects of our world are 'objects' – the It. Others are 'subjects', the fully human (or divine) Other – the Thou. This is a phenomenological observation by Buber. Humans divide the world fundamentally into Others-like-themselves and Objects. However, it is also an ontological observation – this is at the heart of what it is to be human. We address others as either Thou or It. In doing the first, we acknowledge the profound unity we have with them as fellow-beings; in doing the second, we treat others as objects. The former warrants what Heidegger terms 'concern'; the latter, 'use'.

Buber's second claim is that the relationship is not subsequent to the existence of individuals. Relationships pre-exist individuals. This claim is both ontological – the nature of Being – and psychological. We only become individuals through our relating. We do not begin to exist until we have related. This I read as wholly congruent with Rogers' view. The organismic valuing process of the new-born expresses itself not just in terms of needs or drives, but in terms of seeking out the satisfaction of the need for positive regard, in relation to others.

For Buber, therefore, the primary words I–Thou and I–It are both more primitive and more basic than the concept of the isolated individual. It is only possible to live by negotiating the tensions between the two ways of relating. This again parallels Rogers' (1980) key notion that therapy – and indeed all of life – is a way of being. It is appropriate and inevitable that we have relationship that are I–It, but what constitutes our humanity is our unique ability to form I–Thou relationship.

Buber's third point is again deceptively simple on the surface. The relationships embodied in the primary words are not themselves objects. They are not entities. Primary words do not point to things that might exist independently of them. They are performative words. They resemble words like 'I marry you'. They actually achieve what they say in the act of saying. An I–Thou relationship comes into being when, metaphorically speaking, I say 'Thou' to another human being.

This is a dramatic claim. It means that I come into being as a fully existing human only as I learn to say and therefore perform I–Thou relationships. These relationships have a number of fundamental qualities. They are ethical – we offend against *Thous* but not *Its*. They subsist in our having language, just in the way that conditions of worth subsist in our being able to hear the IF of their conditionality in the spoken word. Therefore, the quality of an I–Thou relationship is intimately linked with the language we use and have available to us. The Thou-ness which is innate only comes into being as we contact the world into which we are born.

The consequences of this last point fascinate me. My late friend and colleague, Canon Roger Hooker, was intimately well versed in Hindi and Sanskrit language, thought and literature. Roger argued that the everyday language of relationship with God that some Christians use in a frankly trite way works well enough in English, but that the obvious word in Hindi to translate 'relationship' was what Buber would have termed an I–It word. It stood for the relationship of a cup to a table, said Roger. The notion of I–Thou needed better translation than it often got. He even queried whether the English word 'relationship' could be fully rendered into Hindi. The language that we use deeply influences the world we create for ourselves.

It is not the case that I–Thou corresponds to people-relationships, and I–It to thing-relationships. (Life is not that simple!) People can be treated as objects. However, inanimate objects can also be accorded an I-Thou relationship. Buber cited a benign example of this: the artist is in an I-Thou dialogue with the work of art (Buber, 1958, pp. 22–4). (I will use this as a worked example below.) However, the mirror image of the benign example is important in therapy. I suggest that Buber invites us to consider alcohol as a person in Hannah's life. It not only has a function, but inhabits her world as a friend.

In his essay, 'The Question to the Single One', Buber extends the idea of the I–Thou (Buber, 1961, chapter eleven). He notes that our ability in adult life to create an I–Thou relationship involves detaching ourselves from an identification with the masses, society, culture, the They. What happens as we become Single is somewhat surprising. We need to let go of the idea that truth exists 'out there' and so is to be sought out and possessed by us. Truth, personal truth, is to be lived. We construct truth for ourselves. This does not mean that all knowledge becomes hopelessly relative. Rather it points to the fact that the human or existential notion of truth is ineluctably subjective, and that objective truths, like that truths of natural science, do not count to our existing.

This is again a difficult idea. However, it can be readily linked to some basic concepts in Carl Rogers' thinking. Incongruence manifests itself when we place our locus of evaluation – the way we estimate ourselves to be – in others rather than ourselves. In doing this, we give away our personal power. Conditions of worth, which are by definition external to our organismic selves, are experienced as possessed truths, out there in the world and requiring our compliance, even our allegiance: 'I have always believed that I was set on earth to look after others and not myself. Now I feel that it is not like that at all.' A person who can say this has grasped her task of living out her truth rather than of complying with others' truths that she must possess, and that must possess her.

This internalization of the locus of evaluation, with the consequent relativization of truth can be disturbing. It leaves us with more responsibility, for we have regained our power. That can feel tough, scary as well as good. It can cast a shadow on how we contact our beliefs, such as a religious faith, which we often perceive as 'truth out there', and a much valued truth. It can be experienced as selfish. This latter point is well addressed by David Brazier, who argues that as we regain our personal power, our ability to care for ourselves, we also gain the ability to be genuinely selfless, altruistic, rather than just driven, scripty (Brazier, 1993, p. 27). Letting go of possessed truth in favour of lived truth is disturbing. When clients experience a shift in their locus of evaluation, they need support to begin to live out new experience in the face of the fear of freedom and responsibility (Mearns, 1994a, chapter twenty).

Buber's concept of the I–Thou relationship is radical. In the next two sections, I will invite the reader to check out her grasp of the I–Thou through Buber's own example of the work of art, and then consider some key points of its application to therapeutic practice.

## A Work of Art

Even if the man to whom I say *Thou* is not aware of it in the midst of his experience, yet relation may exist. For *Thou* is more than *It* realises. No deception penetrates here; here is the cradle of the Real Life.

(Buber, 1958, p. 22)

I would say that every true existential relationship between two persons begins with acceptance.

(Buber in dialogue with Carl Rogers, in Kirschenbaum and Henderson, 1990b, p. 60)

In Buber's words can be heard echoes of Rogers' idea of the Good Life and of the core conditions of relating. Buber adds an important perspective to Rogers. He helps me both understand and feel new perspectives on relating. Because the I–Thou is so bound up with human relationships, it is useful to be able to conceptualize a person-to-object relationship as being essentially I–Thou (Buber, 1958, pp. 22–4).

---

**Personal Focus 10.1    Checking the experience of I–Thou**

*The following is based upon Buber's own reflections, but simplified.*

Imagine that you are struggling to create a work of art. What would that be for you? A painting? Music? Sculpture? Even food? It does not have to be 'good' or professional, but just a way of expressing who you are. You are relating to you. As you actively imagine this object that stands for you, let your mind be prompted to perceive what you are doing in making a creation to which you truly relate.

   - When the material flows through your hands, how do you recognize that it is what you want it to be? What in it corresponds to you?
   - When the material is stubborn, and has a will of its own, what in it resists what in you?
   - When the work is true, in what of it can you say: here I see my self?
   - When you see yourself in what you make, do you feel that you have taken a risk? What is that risk? How and where do you feel it?
   - Every time you work, what you make can be different. There are endless possibilities. But you are the Single One. In committing a part of yourself to your work, what do you sacrifice? What do you offer up?
   - When the work is complete and bodies forth what it needs to, what do you recognize?
   - When you look, or when you make, what is the conversation? What have you drawn forth from raw matter?

---

Sometimes, children have an instinctive grasp of the Thou-ness of objects. Perhaps it is part of the quality of play that adults all too readily surrender to so-called 'reality'. The following story is related by the spiritual director, Francis Dewar:

---

**Box 9.1   A story: what emerges**

A father took his young daughter to a friend who was a sculptor. On the first visit, the girl was interested by the sculptor's tools, and by the block of stone on her workbench. But soon the interest passed. On the second visit, she was entranced by the lion's head that had been carved, so lifelike. After a while of looking and touching from various angles, the girl looked up at the sculptor and asked, wide-eyed: 'But how did you know it was in there?'

---

## Saying 'Thou'

One of the simplest applications of the thinking of Martin Buber, for me, has been as a piece of internal dialogue. From time to time I will struggle to see or feel the client to be a human being just like me. I want to objectify her, sometimes because her actions have been difficult or unacceptable, and at other times because I feel fear or apprehension before her and defend myself by rendering her less than fully human.

When this happens, I find it effective to say inwardly, as I look at her or think about her: Thou! This invokes for me, as a mantra, all that Buber means by Thou. Try this for yourself. Such internal speech acts can be powerful correctives of our failure to accept others.

However, there is a problem in this with meaning. Nick Crossley (1996) in his excellent book on intersubjectivity, commends Buber, but then adds,

> My exposition of Buber (1878–1965) must begin with a major qualification. *I and Thou* (1958) is as much a theological work about our relations with God as a philosophical work about intersubjectivity. It is based in the author's faith. I do not share the author's faith, however, and whilst I find the book fascinating with respect to the question of (worldly, material) intersubjectivity, I achive this only by ignoring the theological component. Therefore my (atheistic) reading of Buber necessarily ignores much of what he argues. Indeed it completely misses the point as he presumably intended it. The reader must decide if such exegetic butchery has been worth the effort.
>
> (Crossley, 1996, pp. 10–11)

Indeed Crossley misses the point, but not, I believe, in the way he recognizes. It is a matter of empathic understanding of Buber. I happen to share Buber's faith. I presume – with all the hazard of that presumption – that when Buber likens the human Thou to its origin in the divine who is both Thou and says Thou, then I have at gut level an understanding of the magnitude of Buber's claim. I need to feel the awe in order to understand. Crossley does not need to share Buber's faith, but he cannot excise it in the way he seems to. He needs to struggle within himself to find a version of Thou which he can mean (a)theologically, but which also does justice to the awe in Buber's Thou.

When you say inwardly of another human being this corrective Thou, which strives against our rejection of the other, make sure that it is, as you might say, divine enough.

## The Internalized Other

In moments of pressure, the counsellor will often be founding pondering: What would my supervisor do? This is true for mature and for inexperienced practitioners alike. It is more than a logical or rational question. It is a short-cut to some felt-sense of the way forward. The 'answer' tends to emerge swiftly and with some confidence. It is as if we carry part of the trusted other within ourselves. An internal version of the good supervisor is, as it were, an active principle for reflection. This goes beyond a mere memory of what she or he did in fact say. It is a sense of what he or she *might have* said. The internal supervisor is a functional aspect of the self.

In a similar way, clients carry a version of their therapist within themselves. At the heart of this is the ability of the therapeutic couple to relate to each other. It is the encounter which is internalized (Schmid, 1998). Mick Cooper (2005) argues convincingly that clients relate to themselves as 'Me' – an internal version of Buber's Thou – and as 'Self' – an internalized self-objectification, with the self as an It.

This is a powerful observation by Cooper. It suggests that the client and therapist together work in relationship until the client can relate to herself in an I–Thou fashion. Thus, work with configurations of self (see Chapter 5) might aim to establish a truly interpersonal rather than objectifying dialogue between aspects of the self. From the client's point of view, it could be put like this: When I learn to relate to you (the therapist), I learn in the end to relate to myself as well. Below, in my reflection upon my work with Hannah, I notice that I felt pulled into rescuing her through being the friend that she longed for. (I did not fall for this rescue-act, but sometimes the pull can feel strong.) Yet, the truth was that Hannah's need for befriending was internal. She needed to be a Thou (or in Cooper's terms a Me) for her I.

From time to time I have asked the client to imagine himself as a child, in the hope that this might provoke some sense of compassion, internally. In working with Nicholas, I faced a young man in his late teens for whom his child was not good news. When he eventually pictured his child, the lad was bullied and soaked in urine. The picture revolted Nicholas. It was only in making some contact with this figure of disgust that Nicholas was able to locate some sense of an adult position from which he could offer love and respect to this other being whom he used to be.

## Into Practice

- Listen to the *quality* of the client's language. Does it have an I–It or an I–Thou feel to it to you? How is the client impacting on you? I recall a client who said to me: *I've tried everything except coke* (i.e. cocaine). *She's too beautiful a lady.*
- If you have some sense of the relational quality of your client's language, how are you going to check this out? It is not easy. One way is to look for metaphors – yours or preferably your clients – that have the same relational quality: *It feels for you as if your son just sees you as a coat hanger for his insecurities.*
- When you can see that your client tends to construe some relationships as I–It relationships, what do you feel? (Counter-transference?) Let yourself *feel* the judgement you would like to pass on your client. We can never accord the core conditions unless we allow ourselves to experience fully our desire to withhold them. If you feel judgemental, use supervision to work out whether this is 'your stuff' or whether this is how your client gets others to feel as well.
- When you sense that the client has an I–Thou relationship with alcohol, for instance, check out your responses, as above. Judgemental? About what? How do you experience your client using this relationship?
- When an object is accorded an I–Thou relationship, where in all this is intimacy? Avoidance? Displacement? Replacement? Does your client seek intimacy, or want to avoid it? How are you going to check this out? You could be wrong.
- If an object like alcohol is treated in an I–Thou way, this is a transference relationship. Rogers sees the point of transference being to work through to the genuine relationship. How might the client begin to work through to a genuine relationship with this object and with a replacement?
- For a while, you and the therapeutic relationship might be the replacement. What qualities will you need to provide?
- As the client changes psychologically, there is likely to be a separation out from the environment. She will move towards becoming what Buber calls the Single One. What will she need to support this?
- You will notice a shift, gradually, in her locus of evaluation. She will begin to evaluate herself rather than rely on others' evaluative opinions. The

move from possessed to existential truth can be stressful. Acknowledge and empathize with signs of this stress. Being an I–Thou person with other people for the first time is tough.

- As a client moves towards a more existential experiencing of truth and a more internalized locus of evaluation, she may well experience cultural and societal conflicts. Be alert to these, and acknowledge them. In her family or culture the client may actually be judged harshly for change. This can be obviously true for minority ethic groups, and for gay and lesbian people, for example. What about issues of class or of simple family ethos?

- Be aware of how you talk, think and feel about your clients, particularly in supervision. I–Thou or I–It? For example, if an ending is difficult, is your client an object that you don't want to lose, or a person with a need to be autonomous?

- Be prepared, when appropriate, to facilitate the client to feel and even converse with other versions of themselves, so that an internal dialogue can be established.

- Be prepared to express congruently the quality of your relationship with the client so that they can wrestle with both their own and your perceptions of that, as a means of discovering for themselves better internal relating. This internal I–Me is not about adequate communication only; it is about the fullness of a relationship.

> I would say that every true existential relationship between two persons begins with acceptance.
>
> (Buber in dialogue with Carl Rogers, in Kirschenbaum and Henderson, 1990b, p. 60)

Hannah the Bully was not an easy person to accept. Yet it was at the heart of our work together that our relationship should be, in Buber's sense above, existential. It is not my task here to set out in detail the work. Rather, as I stand back from it I recognize a number of major relational themes. In trusting the client, person-centred therapists have also to trust the quality of their own relating to that client. Existential change happens in the gaps, intimacies and connectivities that make up a relationship.

I notice that Hannah had an I–Thou relationship with alcohol, but an I–It relationship with her colleagues and juniors. She had learned from her parents that relating was difficult, and that her need for intimacy got squeezed out by her father's absence and her mother's insecurity. To desire intimacy is therefore dangerous for Hannah. It can be kept at bay, or perhaps compensated for, by treating human beings as objects, and by treating alcohol as a friend, and a substitute for social contact.

My task for much of the early to middle part of the relationship was to accompany Hannah in her exploration of the relationships here. I made a sub-contract with her in session seven to maintain this focus, as it became clear to her that this was important for her. I avoided diagnosing. Hannah needed not to 'know' but to experience her relating with others. There was often a mismatch between what she thought she was doing with her colleagues and her felt-sense of the relationship or the colleague. This incongruence functioned as a prompt to Hannah that her strategies for relating were not meeting her own organismic needs.

I had to be prepared to allow Hannah to transfer onto me the relational qualities that she acted out in daily life. I could experience her as a bully; a frightened child who awaited my judgement; a vulnerable child who craved my affection but could not tell me so; a grown-up woman who struggled to maintain a surface; a despondent woman who hated herself and whenever the chemical anaesthesia wore thin awaited my judgement of her. I experienced myself as on a roller-coaster of roles and emotions. Above all, I knew that I was not a good-enough substitute for alcohol. I was a false friend, because I encouraged her to feel.

To move towards a genuine-Richard took time, risk and trust on both our parts.

There were moments when I fantasized that I would like to solve her problem by finding her a real friend – for she is actually a lovely person – or even in becoming that friend. (I only need to substitute the word lover for friend to recognize how abuse of clients can arise not just from counsellor lust but from transference and good intentions.) Problem-solving is a false track. Hannah's problem with intimacy emerged in the outside world, but it was rooted in her own being.

Hannah feared her Free Child because it had been so often punished either with rebuke or desertion. She was therefore committed to projecting her fear of rejection by inducing it in others. This was her bullying. Since she dared not be Free Child, she would lock others into a Critical Parent–Adapted Child gameplay. Alcohol provided not just pain-control, but also 'friendship' without the risk of intimacy. Yet she craved that which she denied herself.

All these events are internal to Hannah. Over a period of time empathy, a befriending by me of all of these aspects of her led her to be able to befriend those parts of herself. The move from transferring the befriending role onto me to owning it for herself was slow and fear-ridden. Existential truth is hard to own, as is internal evaluating. It actually is painful. It is a doing of the forbidden. For a while the parental punishments reappear and may be acted out as well as experienced.

I–Thou is enacted within the self as well as socially. Each feeds (or damages) the other.

Martin Buber's construct of relating as either I–Thou or I–It has provided a preliminary vehicle by which to begin to explore the existential element of person-centred therapy. It has proven both practically useful and fairly well self-contained. The next chapter will open up broader issues about the consequences of an existential commitment.

# Further Reading

## *Martin Buber – Primary Texts*

Buber, M. (1958) *I and Thou*. Edinburgh, T. & T. Clark.
Buber, M. (1990) 'Martin Buber' in H. Kirschenbaum and V.L. Henderson (eds) *Carl Rogers: Dialogues*. London, Constable, pp. 41–63.

A good point to begin for most people is with the dialogue with Carl Rogers (Kirschenbaum and Henderson, 1990). This gives a flavour of Buber's way of thinking and Rogers' respect for this. I am ever puzzled as to whether finally Rogers understood why Buber thought that they did not agree on the issue of confirmation of the other person. This is therapeutically an important issue to wrestle with. *I and Thou* is the key text, and expresses most of what matters therapeutically about Buber's intersubjective philosophy.

## *Martin Buber – Secondary Text*

Friedman, M.S. (2002) *Martin Buber: The life of dialogue*. London, Routledge (4th edition).

This is all that you could need about Buber's thought. Buber himself much admired earlier editions of this book. It sets the main theme of dialogue in the context of Buber's life, philosophy and faith. Chapters 10–14 are of particular importance.

## *Existentialism*

Cooper, D.E. (1990) *Existentialism: A Reconstruction*. Oxford, Basil Blackwell.

A good modern introduction to existentialism, but rather quirky in that the author outlines what is typical about existentialism, when nothing is! The way of thinking is diverse. Still, it is a useful way in.

Macquarrie, J. (1972/1991) *Existentialism*. Harmondsworth, Pelican/Penguin.

By far the best introduction to the subject, by the greatest proponent of existentialist philosophy and theology in Britain. The book is still available second-hand. A more refined and balanced approach than Cooper (1991).

Tillich, P. (1952) *The Courage to Be*. New Haven, Yale University Press.

An unusual contribution first made in the early days of the existentialist heyday. Tillich's way of conceptualizing existential anxiety is therapeutically useful. The book is for some also an inspiring read. However, chapter 3 on so-called 'pathological anxiety' should be taken with a pinch of salt. Tillich was not a clinician!

## Existential Therapy

Cohn, H.W. (1997) *Existential Thought and Therapeutic Practice*. London, Sage.
Cooper, M. (2003) *Existential Therapies*. London, Sage.

Two excellent and straight-forward introductions to existential therapy. Cooper (2003) is particularly useful in that he has a firm grasp of, and training in, both the existential and person-centred approaches.

Spinelli, I. (2007) *Practising Existential Psychotherapy: The Relational World*. London, Sage.
Van Deurzen-Smith, E. (1997) *Everyday Mysteries, Existential Dimensions of Psychotherapy*. Hove, Brunner-Routledge.

Two contrasting styles of existential thinking and therapy. In brief, Spinelli is very close to person-centred therapy, with a strong stress on phenomenological tracking of the client, while van Deurzen Smith is closer to the role of a consulatant philosopher.

Yalom, I.D. (1989) *Love's Executioner and Other Tales of Psychotherapy*. Harmondsworth, Penguin.
Yalom, I.D. (2002) *The Gift of Therapy: Reflections on Being a Therapist*. London, Piatkus.

Yalom is ever and always delightful, informative, inspirational and very much himself.

# 10

# The Existential Dimension:
# An Ignored Resource of
# Person-Centred Therapy

The work of Martin Buber falls clearly within the great twentieth-century tradition of existentialist philosophical thought. Because Buber's thinking is so clearly crystallized around the theme of relating, his work is easily available to person-centred theorists. However, beyond Buber lies an ocean of difficult thinking.

It is not possible to give even a minimal account here of existentialist thinking, such is its breadth and diversity. It is not so much a matter of getting a quart into a pint pot, as a gallon into a thimble. This chapter will then begin with Mearns' notion of the existential self; will raise the basic nature of practical, existential thinking through the case study of Tony; will develop and illustrate the concept of existential life-commitments; and finally, will relate the theory to practice through the case study of Heather. I will then elaborate on the meaning of genuineness as an existential commitment through the thought of Emmanuel Levinas and Eugene Gendlin.

## The Existential Self

> The reason for meeting the client at relational depth is that at that intensity of relating the client may give us invited access into his existential Self. He is giving us access to his innermost feelings and thoughts about his Self and his very existence. He is not giving us a false picture layered with conscious defences and pretences – he is including the therapist in the inner dialogue he has within himself. More than that, he is including the therapist in the moment-to-moment discoveries he is making about his Self while he is at the very 'edge of his awareness'.
>
> (Mearns, 1999, p. 125)

In his important article on the configurations of the self, Mearns (1999) is concerned with the way different parts of our selves interrelate. The seeds of this aspect of his thinking are to be found in his work with 'Elizabeth' (Mearns, 1994a,b). While many person-centred theorists have remained suspicious of referring to unconscious thought-processes – the ghost of Sigmund Freud – Mearns relies heavily upon the thesis that the client 'contains' a number of configurations of the self. These somewhat resemble John Rowan's (1990) subpersonalities. These may be seen as particular aspects or facets of our selves which act largely unconsciously as subsystems with a degree of independence and so can communicate with each other or the outside world. Alternatively, they could act as dramatized metaphors for aspects of the self, so that work with configurations of the self is a sort of person-centred dramatherapy. However Mearns' thesis is to be seen, it is clear that he is working in a way that allows clients to invite the therapist to share in depth with their relation to themselves. Mearns calls this the *existential* self. It is key for him that this is not consciously defended. At this level of relational depth, the client has given up trying to fool or deceive the therapist, even by judicious editing of herself.

In the previous chapter, we saw that existentialism is a particular way of thinking about the self; we saw that it was important to have some grasp of this in order to understand Martin Buber and his view of relating as the primary human activity. To understand Buber, it was useful to grasp the existentialist thinking which he did.

Mearns raises the question of the existential self in a new and testing way, that of relating at depth (Mearns and Cooper, 2005). What is an 'existential self'? The word 'existential is open to much abuse. It can be used very loosely. The phrase 'the existential self' can just refer to those deep values and feelings which comprise that nebulous concept 'who we really are'.

A tighter meaning of existential refers to what it truly is to be human. Philosophers throughout the ages have come up with a number of key statements about what it is to be human. Prior to the dawn of the modern age, being human was often seen in terms of relationship to God (as indeed it still is for Buber). René Descartes saw the human as essentially a thinking, eternal consciousness. Plato had seen the human as an immortal soul able to participate in the eternal essences which are the true reality behind the veil of material existence. Existentialist thought, while deeply divided about God, rejects both Descartes and Plato. In the aphorism of Jean-Paul Sartre: 'Existence precedes essence' (Sartre, 1996, p. 29). This means that we construct who we are in our acts of living. We 'exist'; we come to stand out from the world. It is not the case that we are, as Descartes saw us, immutable points of intellect who have being as non-finite essences. It is in the everyday acts of living, of facing our mortality, of being free and responsible, of being and facing anxiety, that we come into being.

It is impossible to overstate the radical effect of thinking in this way. Existentialist thought is not at all easy. Yet, at its simplest, it states that there are both authentic and inauthentic ways of being. Authentic being is to fulfil what it is to be fully human. (Of course, existentialist thinkers come nowhere near to agreeing on what it actually is to be authentic – the content – but there is a large degree of accord that the question of authentic being is at the heart of the human project.) If existentialist thought is anywhere near to correct, then the effect of this on counselling is a major one. It means that the counsellor, in facilitating the client in becoming more fully human, needs to grasp in some way what it is in principle to be fully human. This means, I believe, an understanding in our own experience of human existence. This is an experiential knowledge, but it can also be a philosophical or belief-based knowledge.

As a therapist committed to my own personal development, I need to wrestle with what it is to be, to exist, and to do that wrestling in many modes – thinking, believing, imagining, writing, singing, loving, hoping and so forth.

### Case 10.1 Tony

Tony came to me with a serious alcohol problem. In fact, he was about to enter a detoxification and rehabilitation process. He was in his mid-twenties. In the initial session, he said that his well-to-do mother had given him so much that he wanted. (Father had been off the scene for many years.) He had been encouraged to save, so that, unlike many of his friends, he had a large bank balance after only six or seven years in work. He was deeply ashamed of his drinking. It shamed his family. Yet, as he talked about the money, I realized that he had used drinking to subvert a whole set of his mother's values. I guessed that at heart he was far less materialistic than his mother.

His deep shame at his drinking, and his seeing it as a disease, helped him to find a 'cure'. Detoxification worked. He found a new girlfriend. Life looked up. The content of the counselling seemed riddled with success. Was this Tony, or just the reincarnation of his mother's boy?

After session two, any mention of the money had subsided. It had gone underground. I had a clear hypothesis. For whatever reason, Tony had been deeply dissatisfied with his mother's way of living, her living for money and his conformity to this. The function of drinking had been in part to undermine this. It worked. When he saw me he was pretty broke.

Before we began to work together, fear and self-disgust had led him to want to stop drinking. The old conformity returned, and with it many real and material gains, not to mention his mother's approval. All was well for Tony again.

## Reflection

But what about the money? My hypothesis, my guess, was that he had needed to attack his savings. Doing this had represented something authentic in Tony. This seemed lost now, just as talk of the money had been lost from therapy.

I took the issue to supervision. I identified that I preferred the Tony who attacked mother's materialistic values – but that is about my personal convictions, and certainly cannot be put onto the client. In spite of this counter-transference, I was still left with the question as to who was the more authentic version of Tony. In a time-limited setting, I had to choose. Should I refer back to the money issue in the first two sessions, or not? My supervisor and I concluded that the contract had been to support Tony in quitting alcohol dependency. In a short-term piece of work, it was not my place to take the risk of challenging his authenticity.

I followed my supervisor's advice. I did so with regret and ambivalence. Had I not just colluded with mother and with Tony's conditions of worth to suppress Tony's authentic being again, in the name of cure? I am content that this is the right decision in a time-limited setting in this particular case. The question that it raises is crucial though, and cannot be escaped in long-term work. While I cannot finally know what it is for my client to be authentic, I cannot escape my belief that there is such a thing as authentic being.

However, there seems to be a paradox around the concept of authentic being. In Tony's case, I cannot decide or unduly influence him as to what it is to be authentic. Yet I cannot avoid noticing when I believe that he is not being authentic. This is difficult, slippery. I cannot escape it. Carl Rogers' understanding of authenticity is explored under the phrase 'the good life'.

## Carl Rogers on the Good Life

In 1961 Rogers included in *On Becoming a Person* a paper which he entitled 'A Therapist's View of the Good Life'. He believed that it summarized much of his useful past thinking, now increasingly integrated into his extensive therapeutic practice, about what it is to be a fully functioning human being. This he calls the good life. I intend here to outline some key ideas in the paper to set in context Rogers' use of the term 'existential living'. In so doing, I will suggest that Rogers has limitations as a reflective thinker on existential issues – limitations which person-centred practitioners do well to confront.

Rogers, in this paper, is as ever the phenomenological researcher, who understands the therapeutic process in terms of his own long experiencing of clients. Therefore, the notion of the good life for Rogers is intimately bound up with the question of what would constitute 'optimal therapy':

For the client, this optimal therapy would mean an exploration of increasingly strange and unknown and dangerous feelings in himself, the exploration proving possible only because he is gradually realizing that he is accepted unconditionally. Thus he becomes acquainted with elements of his experience which have in the past been denied to awareness as too threatening, too damaging to the structure of the self.

(Rogers, 1967, p. 185)

Rogers conceives of the good life not as a state, like virtue or contentment or nirvana, but rather as a process. He then characterizes this process as three threads. The first is an increasing openness to experience. The client no longer needs to conceal from herself those elements of incongruence between her self-concept and the world around her. The second is an increasing trust in the organism. The client can trust what she feels and experiences as benign, and liable to lead to self-nurturing behaviours and self-representations. The third is of interest here. Rogers speaks of 'increasingly existential living'.

---

**Box 10.1   What does Rogers mean by 'existential living'?**

- It is to live fully in each moment.
- This happens when people let go of their defences.
- When this happens, each moment is experienced as new.
- The sense of newness arises from the fact that at any point in time the configuration of inner and outer experiencing is unique. It has never existed before.
- Action and experience therefore is sensed as growing out of the moment itself, and not from the conditioned past, nor from the conditioning other.
- Existential living happens when the client feels that 'the self and personality emerge *from* experience, rather than experience being translated or twisted to fit pre-conceived self-structure'.
- Existential living is signalled by loss of rigidity and the imposition of self-structure on experience.

---

I want to say without further ado that I keenly recognize Rogers' categories of experience in the life of my clients and myself. However, this process is just one answer to the question of what it is to live authentically. It may be that the Rogerian answer is necessary to authentic living, but I seriously doubt that it is sufficient.

Rogers does not face the full range of existentialist thought and least of all the darker claims of Heidegger or Sartre to understand authenticity, namely that we are only authentic when we face our mortality and our bad faith in denying our freedom. Rogers' contribution to the question of authentic living is important and psychologically healing, but it makes no pretence to being complete. (For a radical critique of this concept, see Adorno, 2003.)

## Life Commitments

As we have seen in Chapter 9, the necessity to think existentially is rooted in one problem with the phenomenological thinking of Edmund Husserl. Husserl tends to see humans as detachable, perceiving beings, in the end still rather like Descartes' thinking essence, except that perceiving has replaced thinking as the nature of that essence. Existential phenomenologists like Maurice Merleau-Ponty do not see life like this. We are not detachable from life. Rather, we are what we do and make ourselves to be. We are embodied beings.

If this is true, then it is no longer possible to be a mere observer of another human being. We cannot just perceive, however much that perception is born of empathy. We have our commitments. At the most basic, I could not work with a child abuser without his knowing that I am someone who does not at all accept his behaviour. That is my commitment.

The existentialist question is the one set out in relation to Tony. What are my commitments about what it is to be human, to be authentic? They are inescapable. If I cannot hope for people, I should not work as a therapist. My despair will be contagious and harm my clients. I need a grasp of what it is for me to be authentic; beneath this is a frank judgement that some people are committed to their own authentic living, and others are not.

In the next section of this chapter, I will open up, by way of example, two characteristic commitments of existentialist thinking, in such a way that their bonds to the act of therapy can be felt. This selection is bound of course to be personal, biased and incomplete.

These two themes must serve by way of example only. I take:

1. freedom and choice
2. responsibility, anxiety and guilt.

Other themes are for me of equal significance:

- the body and the self
- superficiality and despair
- the courage to exist
- self-estrangement
- faith
- death.

The reader might like to add to this list.

I follow the metaphor of a theme as musical, and set out each theme as an abstract idea, accompanied by a variation, which relates it to the therapeutic context.

## Freedom and Choice

### *Theme*

We are born free, even if, as Karl Marx noted, we are everywhere in chains. We have a deep responsibility to own and take possession of our freedom. To claim and live out our freedom is one key mark of authentic being. This theme is perhaps one that unites existentialists of very different colours. John Macquarrie, an existentialist philosopher and Anglican theologian, writes,

> Existence is authentic to the extent that the existent takes possession of himself and, shall we say, has moulded himself in his own image. Inauthentic existence, on the other hand, is moulded by external influences, whether these be circumstances, moral codes, political or ecclesiastical authorities, or whatever.
>
> (Macquarrie, 1972, p. 206)

We can note how closely this coincides with Rogers' idea of authenticity as the organismic experiencing of life, over against external conditioning. The paradox of this is nicely stated in Macquarrie's idea that we mould ourselves in our own image. Sartre rejects any external authority. Belief or rather obedience becomes for him an act of bad faith (*la mauvaise foi*).

The atheist Sartre and Macquarrie the theologian are surprisingly close to each other. Freedom is at the heart of human existence. It is close to Buber's notion of the I–Thou relationship, in that the ability to see and be seen as a Thou rather than an object is itself constitutive of our being authentically human. Heidegger has real reservations about the degree of freedom we have, over against what he calls fate or heritage, but nevertheless sees freedom as key (Polt, 1999, pp. 102–3). Yet, for me, it is Sartre's concept of bad faith which states the relevance of freedom most incisively:

> You can judge a person by saying that he has bad faith. Since we have defined the human condition as a possessing of free choice, without excuses, without rescue, every person who seeks refuge behind the excuse of their own emotions and passions, every person who invents a determinism is a person of bad faith.
>
> (Sartre, 1996, p. 68)

For Sartre, authentic living is about the ability to claim our freedom in terms of making a choice. At the heart of Sartre's version of freedom and choice is the refusal to renounce choice by vesting it in external loci of evaluation. Moreover, liberty for Sartre is a goal in itself. Freedom *is* authenticity: 'The actions of people of good faith have the quest for liberty in each and every aspect as their ultimate meaning' (Sartre, 1996, p. 69).

Sartre's view is open to a major criticism. There is something capricious about his version of freedom. Whatever choice is made, as long as it is owned as one's own responsibility, is authentic. Eric Matthews points out that this is ultimately a highly individualistic version of freedom (Matthews, 1996, p. 77). We are also social animals, and indeed socially construct ourselves. Therefore ultimate concern may be a more grounded and shared pursuit than this. While I would agree with Tillich that existentialism needs to keep a balance between loneliness and belonging, Sartre's clarity and starkness concerning our self-responsibility is worth facing.

## *Variation*

That which constrains freedom looks to be agreed upon – in part at least – by Rogers and existentialist thinkers. Our freedom is constrained by our social conditioning. Existentialist thinking about freedom complements Rogers' notion of conditions of worth as causing us to exteriorize our locus of evaluation. Sartre and Rogers alike make the plea that we should evaluate ourselves autonomously.

The fact that our need to reject bad faith is an existential commitment alerts me to an aspect of myself, which is crucial. It can be framed as a dilemma. Am I willing, in the name of the client's autonomy, to permit actively that the client should choose to remain an inauthentic being?

This is not a straightforward question, because I can never finally know what it is for another to be authentic. If I fool myself that I do, then paradoxically I will invite them, even unconsciously, to locate their evaluative processes in my own judgements. And yet as soon as I see their renunciation of external evaluation, their leaving behind of their conditions of worth, as a movement towards a healthier functioning, then I can be seduced into insisting that they be free.

Let me put flesh on these bones. Black people and gay and lesbian people, for example, will experience society as making unreasonable demands upon them. If these demands are totally introjected, they become fully operative conditions of worth. But what of the black person who says inwardly that it is too dangerous to be black in British society? How might we respond to a *decision* to remain responsive to others' judgements in this way?

I need to be committed to personal freedom, to personal power, so that I can have faith in my client. But freedom is not an abstract idea without content. I know, I believe, I imagine that I can think what it is to be free for others. That is a sort of empathy. It is also my frame of reference and my prejudice.

I need to believe in the client's freedom actively. I need to be suspicious of my motives. Existentialist thinking helps me to own the fact that freedom is not value-neutral; and that I cannot escape my own personal commitments. I can do no more than examine them in supervision.

## Responsibility, Anxiety and Guilt

*Theme*

Because we are responsible for the way we use our living and our freedom, we are always open to a falling, to use Heidegger's word. Existential guilt is different from either the neurotic guilt of which Freud speaks or the rational guilt of moral responsibility. Neurotic guilt is located in an erroneous evaluation of ourselves, under the pressure of the superego, or similar. Rational guilt is a taking ownership of the wrongs that we do in life, and so is open to forgiveness rather than cure. Existential guilt comes under neither category (Cohn, 1997, p. 72).

Existential guilt is a universal experience of being human. As responsible beings we have before us a range of possibilities. We do not, however, and cannot, live up to these possibilities. We fall short. Macquarrie explains the matter with elegance:

> There is ... something like a tragic conception of guilt among the existentialists. From the very way he is constituted as a finite being who is also free, man is placed in the possibility of guilt, and his 'rising' seems to be inseparable from his 'falling'. In Heidegger the very notion of guilt receives a strange, pre-moral and ontological sense. In German, the word *Schuld* can mean either 'guilt' or 'debt'. In his interpretation of guilt Heidegger makes much of the notion of *Schuld* as debt or lack. In his very being, man is characterized by a nullity or lack of being, and it is upon this basis of nullity that he must take up responsibility for his being.
>
> (Macquarrie, 1972, p. 203)

Guilt, in other words, is the anxiety that we are all capable of feeling in the face of our inability to fulfil the possibilities of our own existence. Yet this guilt is not necessarily negative, even though it may be unpleasant. To feel existential guilt may be to face the fact that I am called to live authentically.

I am clear that, as a matter of fact, Rogers does not deal with existential guilt. In Kirschenbaum and Henderson (1990a) the word guilt receives seven indexed references in Rogers' work. All are about the client facing feelings which they believe to be unacceptable, saving the last which warns the therapist not to reinforce guilt in her presuppositions about the client's motives for coming to therapy (Kirschenbaum and Henderson, 1990a, p. 498). For Rogers, trained as he was in psychodynamic therapy, guilt retains its basically Freudian nature. It is an experience of introjected values together with an awareness that the client has failed these values. Guilt signifies an externalized locus of evaluation. Indeed, the more scholarly secondary texts on Rogers – for instance Barrett-Lennard (1998) and Bozarth (1998) – make no indexed reference to guilt.

By contrast, Brian Thorne, informed by his religious tradition, wrestles with the tension between a negative and non-existential view of guilt and a desire to see shame as having a positive aspect to it:

> Anxiety and guilt, in short, make it impossible for us to be anything other than fearful creatures dreading the future and regretting the past.
>
> (Thorne, 1998, p. 48)

> The basic trouble with human beings is that they cannot trust that they are so constituted that they need not be anxious about their sexuality, their survival or their death.
>
> (Thorne, 1991, p. 79)

It is clear that Thorne struggles to give credence to shame, but rejects the idea that guilt may be in some ways functional. I would like to agree with the second of these quotations. From a Christian perspective, perhaps people may not *need* to feel guilt. However, from an existential perspective, they do in fact feel guilt. That is the human condition.

## Variation

The issue here is how to understand a client who may well not at all understand themselves. Yet the level of not understanding is such as to threaten the very identity of the person-centred therapist.

It is reasonable to suspect that the majority of clients who report feelings of guilt fall under the Rogerian category of self-judgement. The core conditions within the therapeutic relationship will move them in the direction of self-acceptance. Yet once it is seen that there are two other possible meanings of guilt, then this fact becomes also a matter of clinica judgement.

By contrast, some people will feel guilt because of what they have done. They are finally responsible for owning their rational guilt. Self-acceptance and a good therapeutic relationship might well help them to move in the direction of sifting the neurotic from the rational guilt.

This distinction will threaten the role and self-image of some person-centred therapists. It means, as we listen for this distinction, that we need to face the possibility of taking responsibility for our own rational guilt. It also means facing the fact that on some occasions the role of the therapist might move in the direction of secular confessor. For some therapists, this possibility will be feared and denied. Yet client autonomy requires of us an acceptance of rational guilt too.

By contrast with moral guilt, existential guilt is, as Sartre points out, tragic, absurd and inescapable, just because we must choose some possibilities over others, and that without any objective justification (Cooper, 1990, p. 144).

If we see this guilt as unpleasant, tormenting, but part of authentic being, then we must not shirk being prepared to listen carefully for it in clients.

On occasions, I will invite a client to face the dilemma of the nature of their guilt in these very terms. It feels risky. Yet if guilt is part of our being as humans, and all of our being is part of our frame of reference, can the therapist risk not listening for existential guilt? Irvin Yalom writes,

> But the existential concept of guilt adds something even more important than the broadening of the concept of 'accountability'. Most simply put: one is guilty not only through transgressions against another or against some moral or social code, but *one may be guilty of transgression against oneself.*
>
> (1980, p. 277)

To persist in externalizing one's evaluative processes may indeed be a transgression against oneself.

## Into Practice

Existentialist thought bids the therapist clarify both practice and theory. As a practitioner, I carry within me a number of concepts of what it is to be authentic. I acknowledge that it is the client's right as an autonomous human being to decide upon their own criteria for authentic living, but I note that I cannot escape my fundamental commitment that clients benefit from seeking to be authentic, to exercise freedom and choice. Similarly, I note that while clients need to make their own moral and ethical choices, I carry within me inescapable views about the nature of guilt. Once I have seen that some guilt is rational, some existential and some neurotic, I cannot look at any client's guilt feelings without processing what I see against my own awarenesses and belief systems.

In matters of existential concern, bracketing is difficult. It is not a matter of bracketing out my own responses to life's questions. I can do that, by and large. What I cannot bracket out are the questions themselves. This is the existential dilemma for person-centred therapy.

However, beyond this dilemma is a resource. I explore this through the case study of Heather.

---

**Case 10.2   Heather**

Heather has been in therapy for about three years. She had experienced a very impoverished relationship with her father, who, at the emotional level, had consistently walked away from her. She works in a hospice setting. Her concern for the dying and her immense skill in this work is one of the main centres of the power of her living.

Heather has moved through much primitive imagery about her emotional position in life, not least the image of being deep within a pit of isolated and immobile hopelessness. In recent months, her concerns have been far more to do with the spirituality of her work and of her faith. The latter she has had to reconstruct brick by brick. The task is not yet complete.

At a recent meeting, she told of her return from holiday to four dying patients, one of whom she was particularly close to. As she was with the woman, now near death, she recalled looking down and knowing: that is me dying.

I see this single session with Heather in three movements. In the first, we explored the quality of the experience of identifying with the dying one. In the second, we explored how this experience felt both devastating and functional. Heather was able to revisit the echoes of her past. For the first time she made the link within herself between death and desertion in a particular way. She had explored it as a generality in the past. Now it became clear to her that, while the dying of others had mattered so much to her, her fear of her own death was crucial. Her own dying symbolized the cosmic dimension of the desertion theme. Even though she had invested so much in herself, would she finally desert herself in death? Could she with integrity dare to hope in the face of death?

In the third movement, I found myself moving away from my accustomed role of companion in exploring. I offered her the observation that Martin Heidegger had seen death as that which gives meaning to life. As humans, we reflect on life and who we are at a very practical level. We value what we choose. We generate our meanings in this choosing. If life were infinitely long we would have infinite choice. Possibilities would abound, and would therefore be meaningless. In order for our lives to be of meaning, we must have limited possibility. In order to live, we must die.

Heather is a very remarkable human being. What I then observed was an outstanding example of 'self-holding'. Faced with this challenge, she both used me as a sounding board to *think* through what it might mean to her, while at the same time she was able to maintain an awareness of her inner contact with the emotions generated. Her thinking was interspersed with a sophisticated commentary on her own processing.

I felt privileged to witness such an unusual event, and was deeply puzzled about my own transition from companion to fellow-thinker. I had moved, it seemed to me, from Rogers to Socrates, from attending to contending. Why?

The person-centred therapist aims to meet the client in relational depth. Empathy is the struggle to understand. The usual focus of this struggle is the client's world. However, there are times when the deepest human commitment is to be with another human being in puzzlement about the whole world, the nature of being. The deepest way, I had intuited, to be with Heather was to share in her puzzlement. We had by then a marked respect for, and knowledge of, each other. We were by then primarily two human beings who shared in the facing of mortality. The perspective of Heidegger is important to me. It challenges me. I wished above all to share this challenge.

Why might this risk be worth taking?

I offer the hypothesis that the existential element of life is to be shared between therapist and client, and that this can be done in new ways when the client is able to attend to her own processing. I suggest that empathy can be conceived of in three stages throughout therapy. In the first stage, the client's primary need is to be heard at the level of affect and narrative. What do I feel and think? As this becomes a secure element in the relationship, some clients at least need to be heard at the level of their processing. How is it to be me from within? The third stage occurs when the second stage can be held and nurtured by the client. The therapist holds the role of a fellow-traveller in a striving to comprehend being and living. How is it for us to face life as joy, as dread, as responsible, as mortal?

At the point when the client is so functional that they can hold and nurture their own processing, the therapist is freed to hold the position of existential doubt and hope. As the client can feel themselves processing at a deep level, without dependence on another human being to cope with that, then the therapist becomes the Other for a while, the essential Thou with whom the challenge of being can be explored.

Moments such as those with Heather may be rare in person-centred therapy. Even so, there will be glimpses of this at earlier stages in therapy. While the existential therapist may choose to engage in this way for much of the time, the person-centred therapist needs to wait to be invited to engage at this level.

The existential perspective is an immense challenge to person-centred practice. As practitioners, we are to engage with the whole of ourselves in our relating. What is healing is the offering and receiving of the I–Thou relationship. The deeper I enter into relating with another human being, the more of my own life commitments I risk. It is certainly not my place as a therapist to encourage others to take on board my own particular variety of life commitments, nor is it my place to judge theirs. However, I cannot avoid meeting in others the range of concerns that might be held together under the theme of authenticity. Near the end of therapy, and working at existential depth, it may even be that I am invited, as with Heather, to move into something of a more Socratic role. The purist may balk in particular at this last thought. I raise the issue as one that needs far more consideration than it has received to date within the person-centred movement.

## Beyond the Existential

Existential thought challenges us to engage as fully as possible with the client as a creator of meaning. While the concept of genuineness is open to criticism (Adorno, 2003), it remains crucial that therapists should be able to engage clients, from time to time, in active consideration of what it is to be genuine. In this final section, I intend to point to two thinkers who address the very depths of genuineness, but from very different starting points. Emmanuel Levinas invites us to see ourselves as being genuine only when we can see in others the absolute otherness of being, and thus the goal and centre of all our moral commitment. Eugene Gendlin invites us to see the generation of meaning as a natural part of our being in our bodies. These two thinkers seem to be a long way apart, yet each, for me, contributes an indispensible element to the existential quest.

In Chapter 9, I suggested that one application of the thought of Martin Buber was for the therapist to be able to say inwardly of the client: Thou. This is a performative utterance (Austin, 1961). That is, the very inward saying of the word 'Thou' that is effective in changing the attitude, the mindset, of the therapist. In the final section of this chapter, I will suggest that the consideration of one particular problem will lead us to another such utterance – Infinite. This will clarify the whole question of acceptance as an existential category.

In his 1998 chapter on unconditional, positive regard, Campbell Purton first of all notes that if we try to offer acceptance on the grounds of the measured or estimated worth of the other person, sooner or later, it will go wrong. The other person will run out of qualities or reasons to be seen as virtuous and hence acceptable. This is what might be called a bottom-up perspective. The other person is checked out empirically for virtue. Not only will this bottom-up process run out of steam, it is in Rogers' (1957a) terms highly conditional. The qualities looked for become the conditions of acceptance. Therefore, unconditional, positive regard cannot be bottom-up; it must be top-down. This means that the reason for accepting others unconditionally is inherent in what it is to be human. It is an existential quality.

Purton points out that this makes acceptance a spiritual quality, about our very existence as humans. We are acceptable not by what we do but absolutely. This is Levinas' Infinite, as we shall see shortly.

Emmanuel Levinas, whom Peter Schmid (2006) has called a hidden resource for person-centred therapy, was a Franco-Jewish philosopher and scholar of Talmud, of Lithuanian extraction. He engaged for almost the whole of the twentieth century with the greatest minds of French philosophy, from Bergson, through Sartre to Derrida. He offers an unusual and, I believe, useful view of being human. His major works (Levinas 1969, 1998) are highly complex, and yet some of his images are accessible. (The image of the face will form an important part of the next chapter, on spirituality.)

One of his key categories is the Infinite. It is not only compatible with the idea of God, but also bears a secular meaning. It is therefore available to all regardless of their religious standpoint. Levinas' starting point is to observe the tendency of Western thought – and he means all of it! – to reduce the whole of life to a totality (*totalité*). The meaning of the totalizing of life needs careful grasping. The idea relates in some ways to the derived word 'totalitarian'. Just as a totalitarian régime reduces the whole of life to the patterns and interests of that regime, just as some Marxist thought reduces all of life to economics, so Western thought ensnares the whole of life in its own categories. All is reduced to what Levinas calls the Same (*La Même*) – that which is evident in life and beyond which there is nothing.

In trying to grasp what Levinas means by this, feelings can be as useful as the intellect. The Same is claustrophobic, and abhors that which it cannot comprehend, cannot enclose in its own system. The Same omits to look beyond itself, but also asserts that it is all that there is, and so the beyond is void, and without meaning. The imagination is thrown back by the Same upon itself, and the images that are obvious in its world. The Same believes that its language is supreme; cannot take into account the fact that other languages offer other views of reality. An everyday example may help. The person who is obsessed by money or possessions can only negotiate life in those terms. The Same therefore has spiritual consequences. When all is reduced to money much that is noble in life is excluded. In a similar way, the Same, in interpersonal terms, reduces all people to be comprehensible by our own categories. It threatens to annihilate the validity of difference.

---

### Box 10.2   The Same and the Infinite

**The Same.** Imagine standing in a beautiful part of the country-
side, where the green fields and blue skies, tinged violet, stretch
to the distant horizon. All that you see is wonderful, delicious.
Yet, in your culture, you have been taught that there is nothing
beyond the horizon. All that there is stands within the grasp of your
vision.
**Beyond?** You begin to doubt what you have learned. The earth is
curved. Beyond the horizon is more. But it is more of the Same. Why
should it differ? It is predictable.
**The Infinite.** You look up. The blue sky is no boundary, and beyond it
there stretches that which is beyond imagining. The Infinite will not
be imagined or imaged. It will not be held within the horizon.

---

The opposite of the Same is not the different but the Infinite (*L'Infini*), that
which is without measure. It is not without measure in a merely technical sense
like five divided by zero. It is immeasurable because it cannot be confined to
the ego, the self, the Same. For Levinas the idea of the Infinite is a ethical one
which counsellors might dwell upon. The Same is self-sufficient; the Infinite
is about mutuality and looking beyond oneself for the satisfaction of need
(*besoin*).

Levinas has a powerful metaphor for this – the caress. A caress might seem
an everyday and predictable thing, yet this is how he invites us to see it:

> The tenderness of skin is the very gap between approach and approached,
> a disparity, a non-intentionality, a non-teleology. Whence the disorder of
> caresses, the diachrony, a pleasure without present, pity, painfulness. Prox-
> imity, immediacy, is to enjoy and to suffer by the other. But I can enjoy
> and suffer by the other only because I am-for-the-other, am signification,
> because the contact of the skin is still the proximity of a face, a responsibil-
> ity, an obsession with the other, being-one-for-the-other, which is the very
> birth of signification beyond being.
>
> (Levinas, 1998, p. 90.)

In his typically difficult prose, Levinas sees the boundary of the skin as that
which gives us access to the other person as one who is not another version
of us, but another world. One of the conditions of encounter is a permit-
ting of the Other to be precisely the Other, and not another edition of the
Same. Why? To caress another is so different from mere touch, which might
be objectifying. Yet, when I caress, I open up my own self to the demands of

the other. Levinas offers us three contiguous words for this ethical relationship: face, responsibility and obsession. To understand the Infinite, we need to imbibe the taste of these words.

What then is it to say Infinite to another, within oneself?

First, it is to know that the other person is connected to me by my ethical obligation to her. Secondly, she is connected to me by my final inability to penetrate the otherness of her, and in particular her ability to be utterly beyond me. Thirdly it is to know that empathy is a limited quality of being. If I am overcommitted to empathy, then I will reduce the Other to the Same, a clone of my ego. Fourthly it is to grasp the very limitation of my understanding as that which moves towards a definition of the other person, and so on. Yet it is practice which is as ever the best illustration.

Let us return to the case study of Heather, above. Heather saw in the dying woman an image of herself. There could have been two versions of this image. If the dying woman was merely the Same, then she would have been nothing more than a reminder to Heather of her own mortality. That would have been objectifying of the woman, and so quite futile as a vista upon herself. It was my experience of my work with Heather that the other was truly the Other, in spite of her words that that is *me* lying there. Heather's compassion reached out to the otherness of the dying woman, to imagine the limitless horizon of her being. Had she reduced her to the Same, then she would have been no more than an object-lesson. She was truly Other, and hence like the otherness of Heather, a proper image of her humanity and her being.

Inwardly say to the client: Infinite. Feel what might be for you the shift in felt-perspective.

Levinas is important but he is difficult. He takes us to places in which meanings feel both important and slippery, all at the same time. In the brief previous paragraph I invited you to consider what it would be to think of your client, and hence of yourself as well, as Infinite. This seems to me to be an act of meditation in which the meaning cannot be *deduced*. It has to be *intuited*, felt. It is in this context that I want to consider the thought of Eugene Gendlin, even though his significance for person-centred therapy goes a long way beyond what this book can do justice to.

Eugene Gendlin was a colleague of Carl Rogers, a friend and companion in scholarship. He is perhaps best known for his procedure known as focusing (Gendlin, 1981; Purton, 2007) – see Chapter 2. However, his earlier and more scholarly study (Gendlin, 1997) dates from 1963, and is a version of his doctoral thesis. In this, he proposes that meaning – and hence being human – is characterized by experience. We *feel* what we mean long before we consciously or systematically *think* it. He puts it thus:

> Meaning is experienced. It is not only a certain relationship between verbal symbols and perceptions. If meaning was only these 'formal' or 'objective'

relationships, our speaking would be like the speech of a phonograph record. A phonograph record may 'obey' all the rules of logic, syntax, and of the objects about which it speaks, yet it has no experience of the meaning of which it speaks. When we humans speak, think or read, we *experience* meaning.

(Gendlin, 1997, pp. 44–5, original italics)

Meaning is developed within us, as a felt-sense of what is. It forms in our bodily sensations before we conceptualize, own or express it. When we are not congruent, these emergent felt-meanings are cut off and repressed. (Gendlin's theory has a very good fit with Rogers' theory in this.) As we learn to pay attention to felt bodily experience, we come to appreciate the meanings, welcome or unwelcome, which we need to generate. Focusing is a process-directive way of facilitating the client in forming the meanings that are latent. We do not need to undertake this procedure in order to find the importance of Gendlin's theory of meaning. Rather we need to be able to listen to what the client may or may not be resisting in terms of meaning.

Let us return to the case of Tony, above, to understand this more. I guess that if I had had time and the contract to persist in therapy with Tony, then we might well have accessed a sense that the waste of money in his addiction felt strangely good, not least because his father so disapproved of it. If Tony had been able to remain with this felt-sense, this apparent contradiction, he could have reached the underlying meaning as I estimate it to be. He could have made a conscious decision to reject his parents' materialism and begin to find what his own life held for him as meaning and purpose. As David Rennie (2006) argues in his consideration of what he calls *radical reflexivity*, we find our true personal power when we realize that in becoming conscious of our self-awareness we have the space, perhaps for the first time, to make our own decisions.

When, therefore, we use the thought of Levinas to say towards a client, Infinite, we are attempting to tap into a sense, a felt-sense of the beyond. This is difficult because it is part of what the modern age in its reductionism relegates to the private and often the contemptible. Levinas' Infinite can echo the religious or the spiritual, even though he maintained at all times that his thought was secular philosophy. We are striving to feel beyond what we habitually do. Yet, only when we can access a felt-sense of a whole range of meanings can we do justice to the existential potential of our clients.

The existential themes of therapy, not least the theme of humans as images of the Infinite, together with Gendlin's observation that all meaning is generated first within the felt-sense, lead on to a growing and major concern of person-centred therapy – its spirituality. This will be the concern of the next chapter. It is an extension of our concern with the existential.

# Further Reading

## General

See the reading list for Chapter 9.

## Levinas

Levinas is advocated by Peter Schmid as a hidden resource for person-centred therapy. However, he is an extraordinarily difficult author to read. Perhaps the best starting points are:

Critchley, S. and Bernasconi, R. (eds.) (2002) *The Cambridge Companion to Levinas*. Cambridge, UK, Cambridge University Press.

Levinas, E. (1996) 'Transcendence and Height' in *Basic Philosophical Writings*, A.T. Peperzak, S. Critchley, and R. Bernasconi (eds.). Bloomington and Indianapolis, Indiana University Press, pp. 11–31.)

Worsley, R. (2006) 'Emmanuel Levinas: Resource and challenge for therapy'. *Person-Centered and Experiential Psychotherapies 5:3*, pp. 208–20.

## Gendlin

Gendlin, E.T. (1981) *Focusing*. New York, Bantam Books.

Gendlin, E.T. (1997) *Experiencing and the Creation of Meaning: A Philosophical and Psychological Approach to the Subjective*. Evanston, Northwestern University Press.

The 1981 book is a good introduction to the technical procedure of focusing. However, the 1997 book is the key to Gendlin's deep insight into the relationship of body-awareness to meaning in life.

Purton, C. (2007) *The Focus-Orientated Counselling Primer*. Ross-on-Wye, PCCS Books.

The most compact and accessible introduction to Gendlin's thought.

# 11

# The Spirituality of Counselling: Phenomenology, Existentialism and Beyond*

Spirituality is a notoriously difficult subject to talk about. The word itself has many meanings, some of which are slippery and deceptive. However, clients – and therapists – increasingly need to talk about spirituality. It is an aspect of their process. This processing is often a form of questing for the beyond, a *cri de coeur* that: There must simply be more than this! Therapy has been a secular and at times even reductionist life view. However, until we can openly understand and refer to the spiritual, we will find that clients obligingly keep it out of the therapy room. *The phenomenological and existential principles which underlie therapy require that we are in tune with this aspect of our clients' processing.*

This chapter outlines one of the ways in which a clear understanding of the phenomenological and experiential nature of person-centred therapy can help the practising counsellor make these links. Without clear understanding, talk of spirituality can degenerate into mere sentimentality or incoherent personal agendas. The first half of the chapter deals with the underlying phenomenological principles which can enable coherent talk of spirituality within the profession. The second half asks how a consideration of the transcendent in particular can help our practical work.

My own spirituality is marked out by images and metaphors which attach a particular value to the space in which the relationship occurs. These include

* This chapter is based on two articles: 'Can we talk about the spirituality of counselling?' *Counselling 12:2*, Rugby, BAC, pp. 89–91; 'More than Meets the Eye.' *Therapy today 19:2*, Rugby, BACP, pp. 34–6. I am grateful to the editor for permission to re-use the copyright material here.

metaphors of the space as play, as parenting, as drama, as presence, as holy. These can be shared, discussed, debated with others. While these feelings, images and beliefs that populate my personal spirituality of counselling are valuable to me, this alone cannot validate their use. Spirituality is a public discipline. I need to *say* something. I need to speak in a way that can be challenged by others. When I can make explicit the links between my experience of counselling and my spirituality then I make myself vulnerable to dialogue with friend and foe alike. We may come to a deeper understanding. Only then am I open to the client *qua* spiritual human being (whatever that might mean to her). *My own spirituality is important to my work, not only because I try and embody all of who I am in therapeutic encounter, but also because I can only understand others' process in this area if I am in touch with my own.*

## Making Links

Carl Rogers was for much of his life a scientific empiricist. He had long ago left not only the mid-American fundamentalism of his mother but also the liberal Christianity of United Theological Seminary, New York. Following his wife's death, he had become interested in the paranormal. At about the same time, he began to identify a transcendent quality in relating. A year before his death, Rogers (1986a) wrote,

> When I am at my best, as a group facilitator or a therapist, I discover another characteristic. I find that when I am closest to my inner intuitive self, when I am somehow in touch with the unknown in me, when I am perhaps in a slightly altered state of consciousness in the relationship, then whatever I do seems to be full of healing. Then simply my *presence* is releasing and helpful.

It has been a matter of debate as to whether Rogers' experience is tinged with the megalomania of one who is losing a grip on life, or whether he recognizes anew, at this point in life, the transcendent in his experience of counselling. The choice is the reader's. I suggest that it is unwise to dismiss too readily the quality of being to which Rogers alludes. Yet it is beyond doubt that Rogers does not find a fully public language for his experience. Hence the uncertainty as to how his followers might view what he had to say. They are divided between seeing his thoughts on the spiritual at the end of his life as a new and important realization of what it is to be human, on the one hand; on the other hand, as an eccentric move and even a betrayal of his commitment to empiricism.

To process further this awareness of the spiritual, a preliminary definition is useful. *To talk of the spiritual is to mark out an event, experience or theme as transcendent. Having performed this act of marking out, only then should we find ways to talk about the 'What?' or the 'How?' of it.*

A metaphor underlying this chapter is that of making a link, drawing a line, between my therapeutic practice and my spiritual experience. Which end of the process of linking do I begin with? I could begin with my spiritual experience or with my therapeutic experience. This is a key methodological issue. I need to ask which is the more basic for me. My fundamental claim is that what I do as a counsellor is of the same sort of significance as what my faith describes to me. As for Rogers so for me, the act of therapy *is* an experiencing of the transcendent. Of course, I cannot prove this claim in a deductive fashion. What I can do is to show that my therapeutic experience is congruent and inductively in tune with my faith. This suggests that I start with the therapeutic. It is basic at the level of experience. I experience therapy as spiritual, and this raises the whole question for me. This is only relevant because my clients experience living as spiritual, even though there would be very great diversity in the expression of this fact. I need to equip myself to hear them that they can feel free to bring this aspect of themselves to therapy.

## Phenomenology as Public Language

When I look at Rogers' comment upon the transcendent nature of the therapeutic relationship I can identify what seems to be a similar experience, but I articulate it differently. I experience myself as working within the theatre of a sacred drama in which the client's presence and mine are a constant surprise and delight to me. I can speak of it being a place of God at work. This is where I need to forge the link. If I can use the language of the sacred arena in more than a sentimental way, it will be because I can offer a common language for both therapy and faith.

*When I am in touch with a client in a way that is effective and healing, phenomenological theory suggests that we, the client and I, are in process of grasping that which is beyond the knowing of either of us.* This is not in itself mystical. The unknowability and our paradoxical grasping beyond it are both aspects of the phenomenological theory of knowledge.

How is this the case? When I explore in experiential and existential depth with a client, we commit ourselves to a new grasping of that which is within the client's awareness (including what might loosely be called the unconscious). Neither of us knows what this is. However, there is always an intuition that it relates to a reality beyond the 'mere' subjective, to the external world as it really is. Sometimes – perhaps always – the quality of what is known is interpreted, marked out, as spiritual, because it is felt to transcend human banality.

It is logical enough to state this *as a fact*, but to experience it is to experience the spiritual. Phenomenology provides the person-centred practitioner with a way of describing in a therapeutically coherent way the beyond-ness of experiencing, in which words and images are always stretched to express meaning.

For some, this is the end of the story. To be successfully grasping the ungraspable feels special. For many others, however, it is not the end of the story. This structure of experience parallels, reflects, forth-tells a deeper structure within reality.

## Phenomenology as Spiritual

When I experience the fact that the client and I are in the paradoxical state of grasping after the unknowable, how does the phenomenological principle help me to understand this as spiritual?

As long as the meaning of 'spiritual' centres upon the self-transcendence of the human subject, then phenomenology has great potential for expressing this. It can be expressed in secular or religious terms.

As I explore with my clients their world-view, their very perception of all that matters to them, I move beyond a need to be accurate in my sharing in that perception. We become aware at some level of the ultimacy that these signify. Even if the belief-content may vary, its ultimacy does not. As therapy progresses, my client may experience herself as more able to make choices. The ultimacy of this is that she is responsible for her own life. She can live in full awareness of her freedom or she can live in what Sartre (1996, p. 52) called 'bad faith' (*la mauvaise foi*) – a false renouncing of her freedom. She can face the fact that her choice is limited and, moreover, limited by virtue of her own mortality. She can note that death gives ultimate meaning to life. She can struggle with the problem that, as conditions of worth and life-scripts gradually recede, she needs to discover what it is to live authentically as herself.

The quest for authenticity in living can be disturbing, frightening. The old, oppressive patterns are often safer, familiar territory. The need to be oneself comes hard. At the very depths, being oneself is a mystery. Can I actively participate as a human being in the fundamental act of Being, in creation and creativity? Or am I safer being only at the behest of others? From secular and religious perspectives, this is a question of deep spiritual meaning, of ultimate concern. As Martin Buber wrote,

> Spirit is not in the *I* but between *I* and *Thou*. It is not like the blood that circulates in you, but like the air in which you breathe. Man lives in the Spirit if he is able to respond to his *Thou*. He is able to if he enters into relation with his whole being.
>
> (Buber, 1958, pp. 57–8)

## Into Practice

The therapeutic relationship is increasingly spoken of as spiritual. Yet, the notion of spirituality is ineluctably vague. People with very different world-views may have similar spiritualities; those with similar experiences and belief-systems may show great spiritual diversity. All I have attempted in a short space so far is to show that the experiences of therapy and spirituality can be linked by a careful consideration of the phenomenological principles that underlie both. The practical question for each therapist, in responding at existential depth, is, am I in touch with my own spirituality? Yet, even the language of this question feels loaded to some. Like Dave Mearns (Mearns and Thorne, 2000, p. x), some people may find it easier to think in terms of their existential depth(s).

---

**Personal Focus 11.1   Am I in touch with my own spirituality?**

- Is there an event or other motif in your life that hints at your ultimate value?
- Is there an image that you have of yourself or of someone else that helps you see them or you as of total and unconditional worth?
- Are there metaphors, pictures, works of literature or other forms of art which express the beyond for you?
- What do you want to do with the rest of your life?
- Sooner or later, you will die. How does this thought and fact affect your view of your being alive?
- Has your view of the last question always been the same or has it changed at all?
- Does God-talk refer to anything for you? Can you make for yourself a mental image or feeling about this?
- Have there been moments in therapy – your own or your clients – when, however vaguely, you have felt in touch with the ultimate or the transcendent, whatever you might mean by this? Be as free as possible about its meaning for you.
- If anyone speaks about the spiritual, what feelings do you have? Longing, fear, hope, dismissiveness, emptiness, love?
- Can you feel or understand the idea that the spiritual is not only a religious idea?
- 'However limited, I am still responsible for my life.' How do you feel about this? What do you believe?
- 'I bring my whole self into the counselling relationship.' What does this mean to you? What feelings do you have?

---

# Meeting Others

> 'When i use a word,' Humpty Dumpty said, in a rather scornful tone,' it means just what I choose it to mean, neither more nor less.'
>
> Lewis Carroll, *Through the Looking Glass*, Chapter VI

There is a tendency in spirituality discourse to behave rather like Humpty Dumpty and make language do just what you want it to. The first half of this chapter has made a case for looking for a shared or public language of spirituality. Yet, this is only a beginning. Through the public language, beyond the phenomenological and existential, is the possibility of people meeting across difference. There are many sorts of difference to cross. There is the difference between a Jew and a Muslim; the difference between what is alleged to be religion and what is alleged to be non-religious spirituality; there is the difference of culture and ethnic heritage. There is the difference inherent in the divergent ways of hearing and feeling metaphor and transcendence. There is a difference between the materialist consensus of the West and those of all traditions who look to see beyond this. There is the difference between people relishing life in diverse fashions (Trivasse, 2004).

When we can develop a public discourse for spirituality, which is the objective counterpart of an inner awareness of our relation to the spiritual, we can meet others at depth. That is to say, we can encounter others in their diverse inwardness and value-sets, in their experience of being human or of being with God or whatever. In this fact, the subject of the spirituality of counselling ceases to be a quirky adjunct to the profession, and becomes one major criterion for thinking about healing. This link is based on the thinking and work of the Austrian person-centred scholar, theorist and practitioner, Peter Schmid. Schmid (1998) argues that healing is based upon encounter with another at depth.

# What Stops Us Meeting?

Throughout the literature a number of problematic themes arise:

---

### Box 11.1　Problems with defining spirituality

- Spirituality is set over against religion, so that the allegedly bad is projected away from the messianic new enterprise of spirituality.
- Anthropology, the theory of what it is to be human, is similarly split into spiritual and non-spiritual components. This violates the principle of holism.
- There is an uncritical presumption that spirituality is to do with peak experience. Carl Rogers headed down this road. Some spiritualities specifically reject the significance of peak experience.

> The discourse within counselling is seemingly deaf to the parallel
> discourses on spirituality in healthcare, education, Christian and
> other theologies, religious studies and multi-disciplinary studies
> in spirituality.

These errors crop up for a number of reasons. The word spirituality is used as a means of dealing illegitimately with what we might call the difference between good and bad religion, however this might be defined. There can be uncritical thinking about peak experience, often rooted in an untenable reification of the spiritual – treating it as if it were a thing, like Plato's or Descartes' idea of the soul. This is made worse when thinking about spirituality in other disciplines is ignored. Counsellors can be very insular. Religion and spirituality, like science, can be kidnapped by individuals' agendas, so that instead of cool thought the writer bombards others with their own programmes, and in particular treat new spiritualities as if they had no religious beliefs inherent in them. All of these can be seen as merely careless or bad practice.

However, there is a viewpoint of the whole issue that suggests that within our societies today there is another and more significant source of pressure. It is this pressure which both distorts and challenges talk of spirituality. It had been a commonplace of the history and sociology of religion that we have been moving, at least in Western Europe, through a process of secularization, in which religion becomes marginalized and privatized. This alleged process had begun nearly 300 years ago with the early Enlightenment philosophers. Alternatively, it began with the process of industrialization and the loss of social cohesion that went with it. (Both accounts are somewhat mythical in my view!) In any case, it seemed to be the predominant culture that religion and all that went with it would fade into oblivion, to be replaced by a new consensus – the secular world-view. In other words, spirituality is seen as the opposite of the rational.

The death of religion or of spirituality has been deeply challenged by the Exeter sociologist of religion, Grace Davie (1994). In her study of religion in Britain since 1945, she concludes that the real state of the nation might be summed up as 'believing without belonging'. If her thesis holds, there is considerable religious and spiritual believing going on, but this is increasingly detached from formal religion. In other words, the myth that we are moving towards a secular consensus holds little water. This might explain the rash of militant atheist diatribes to hit bookshop shelves recently (e.g., Dawkins, 2006). It is maddening that we are not becoming sane and non-religious in a predictable way. At the same time, people seek belief, but in ways that are diverse and at times isolated and privatized.

The discourse of spirituality consequently has two different roles to occupy. It needs, as I have already argued, to put forward a public and to some extent neutral account of why the whole discipline should be taken seriously in counselling. At the same time, it expresses a thirst for the beyond, the simple statement that there must be more. The first role is neutral; the second is committed, but far more warmly human.

*I therefore suggest that spirituality be defined as a seeking for some deep quality of human existence in terms of values, meaning and transcendence.* Human values are not just about being ethical, although that is important. Rather, values are retroflexive: when I express my valuing of some other, I value my own living. Similarly, the role of finding meaning in life has been long recognized in therapy (Frankl, 1987). The word transcendence, however, marks a more difficult aspect of human existence. To transcend is to go beyond, to exceed the obvious. It can be religious or secular. I want to illustrate this elusive quality with two examples:

1. The nature of truth is vexatious. There can be hard, cynical, reductionist version of truth, which detract from life's imaginative and spiritual texture. On the other hand, some claims to truth seem to be without any foundation. How do I keep a rich enough account to transcend reductionism and yet avoid sheer fantasy? It has been suggested to me that truth might be seen as having two 'flavours'. It can be either Likely or Lovely. I need to think (and feel) very hard as to how much of each I need on any occasion. By way of illustration, I am prone as a non-mathematician to see mathematics as about the Likely – 'scientific'. Mathematicians, by contrast, know that the truth is often about the Lovely. A theory that is true can be described as true for almost aesthetic reasons. Even maths touches the spiritual, it seems!
2. A parable. Beyond True and False, there is a field where we may meet. In inter-religious dialogue, in encounter, there must be a reaching of the field which is beyond True and False. My responsibility is to discover the way through to it. If I do not, I am ensnared in True and False, often as an extension of my own ego.

Neither example exactly points to an absolute definition or understanding of the spiritual, yet each stretches language towards the beyond. This is a particular genius of metaphor (Ricoeur, 1975) – to open up the possibilities of existential thinking.

## Transcendence and Metaphor

In a recent, brief study of spirituality and groups (Worsley, 2008b), I suggested that the notion of transcendence could be explored through two particular metaphors: the mirrored box and the face.

The mirrored box is a psychodynamically informed picture of the world as essentially a projection of parts of the self. If I stand in a large box or room, where all of the interior surfaces are mirrored, perhaps in complex fashion,

I can come to perceive the world around me as rich and varied. And yet, all of it is a reflection – projection – of me. This is a claustrophobic, oppressive image. If it is a metaphor for what is, then all is the same and there is no beyond. I, Richard, am ensnared in a world that is, in the words of Friedrich Nietzsche, human, all too human.

By contrast, the metaphor of the face seeks consciously for the beyond (Levinas, 1969, 1998). It comes from the writing of Emmanuel Levinas (see Chapter 10). The human face is a unique object-in-the world. It represents encounter. We speak of meeting face-to-face. Yet, the face invites us to go beyond the surface of encounter. It invites us not just to see someone-like-ourselves, for that is to reduce the whole world to the same, like the mirrored box. It invites us to see the other, or rather the very otherness of the other. It makes a moral demand upon us that speaks of total otherness. We may not reduce the other to a version of ourselves. The otherness of the other is absolute, beyond the mere difference between persons, but a signifier of the immense call upon us from another to recognize the wholly unattainable, uncontrollable, irreducible – alterity. The face, which looks on its surface so much like my face, is the indicator of transcendence.

The previous paragraph may feel to be very testing reading. Such is the difficulty of Levinas' thought. Yet, I value his work precisely because it stretches words. I can, of course, dismiss him as wilfully obscure – I think he is not so – or just plain beyond me. But it is in reading and re-reading him that I have found my imagination fired by this and other images, which bring life to dry words. The metaphor is perhaps the only way to deal with the transcendent, because only the metaphor can seduce us into the total beyondness which spirituality and religion thirst for.

The richness of Levinas' metaphor is that it does two apparently contradictory tasks. It offers a highly abstract version of transcendence, and hence one that is independent of creedal content – for so Levinas argued. However, it also embodies the strong claim that whatever the transcendent might be, it is an essential part of being human. We cannot be human without transcendence. This claim, if it is true, gives us hope, and also demands of us, to build into accounts of therapy the transcendent.

It is not my claim that transcendence is only attainable in practice through Levinas' thought – for that would be a dismal fate! All lively metaphor has this quality to it. In the next section, I want to illustrate this in the work of John O'Donohue.

## Into Practice – Spiritual Wisdom

### The Unknown Companion
There is a presence who walks the road of life with you. This presence accompanies your every moment. It shadows your every thought and

feeling. On your own or with others, it is always there with you. When you were born, it came out of the womb with you; with the excitement of your arrival, nobody noticed it. Though this presence surrounds you, you may still be blind to its companionship. The name of this presence is death.

(O'Donohue, 1997, p. 243)

John O'Donohue, who died in early 2008 at the age of only 52, was a priest and philosopher, who wrote widely on Celtic spirituality. His writing is rooted in the Christian and pre-Christian spirituality of Ireland, a spirituality deeply anchored in nature and in the rhythm of life, often rural and remote life. He lived in the far west at Conamara. His work is at one and the same time profoundly Christian, easily accessible to all, whatever they might believe, deeply informed by continental philosophy, and deeply imbued with the insights of Gestalt therapy. In one of the obituaries written at his death, it was said that O'Donohue displeased those who wanted easy answers. He is perhaps nearer to the true in a proper sense of that word.

Above is one of O'Donohue's more shocking and demanding images – the Unknown Companion. I see him as working within the ancient wisdom tradition. Knowledge is about intuition, contact with the world and the divine, and the right shepherding of life's metaphors. What appeals about his writing is his ability to link together a number of elements: an imaginative grasp of landscape; a sense of the wholeness of lived experience, such as the welcome of a peat fire or a true friend; a locating of this within the lifespan of us all; the rhythm of our living and growing; above all, a sense that the lived moments seek completion, so death is neither a stark curse nor an insipid hope, but a dark and invisible companion to whom we are invited to relate.

In some sense, O'Donohue's faith shines, but it is not oppressive. It shines not because he has answers, but because he focuses the questions. Implicit in this focusing is the sense that life probably makes enough sense to him for his images to hold me while I wrestle. It is the faith of the counsellor in life that holds the client too. When a therapist works with a suicidal client, she really does need to know why *she* wants to be alive.

The metaphors and images in O'Donohue are above all invitations. For example, when I read the image of the Unknown Companion I am invited to face my own mortality. I am invited, though to face it in a particular way. Death is my companion. Is this a grim joke? Or might it be that death may come to me as a friend? Why? Perhaps I do not yet know the answer to this. The challenge is how I will orientate myself to my own death. The image is full of potential meaning. The word *companion* is neither an empty nor a neutral word. Yet, it is not a word that conveys a creedal belief either. I am invited in, to wrestle, as Jacob wrestled the angel, for better or worse.

May you be given wisdom for the eye of your soul, to see this beautiful time of harvesting.

(O'Donohue, 1997, p. 242)

Immediately prior to the image of death as companion comes O'Donohue's key image for ageing – harvesting. Here, I note two qualities. The metaphor is full of content. It is not formally creedal, but full of a trans-creedal faith. To grow old is to harvest. It is to separate the wheat from the chaff. It is to be forgiven and to forgive. It is pregnant with hope in a period of apparent decay or denial. The images and metaphors of spirituality invite us to engage. They are far from value-free. They are laden with meaning, and yet they invite us to find transcendence in our own way.

In therapy, the therapist can sometimes risk offering a metaphor that is exactly like this.

---

**Box 11.2  A group metaphor**

Rachel had found it tough to speak in the group. She had been silent for most of the time, session after session. I sensed that she was not just nervous, but that she felt unworthy to be heard.

The group began in session seven to talk about feelings of guilt that they experienced. It belonged to them, but sometimes it was passed round in the family. A metaphor came to me, a familiar one.

Guilt is like a beach ball, light and large and obtrusive. It can sit on anyone's lap. Suddenly I imaged a ball and threw it to Rachel: Catch! Now throw it back to me! Rachel, how was that for you. In the metaphor and in its sheer physicality she found the power of speech.

---

## But Does the Spiritual Really Matter?

'Humans are spiritual beings.' By now, I hope the reader recognizes that this is a difficult statement, and not one with a single, obvious meaning. For therapists, the challenge of it is this. The quality of being alive that the word spiritual might indicate is present in the therapeutic relationship. There is likely to be therapeutic and anti-therapeutic spirituality. We can encounter others at the level of values and meaning and transcendence, and we can do it more or less well. This means that we can discuss how well we are working in this perspective. It is part of the incoherence of the current discourse that little has been said about this. (We are still trapped in partisanship.) A useful exception to this is the writing of Peter Schmid. He works from the category of encounter.

His work is deeply informed by Emmanuel Levinas. Indeed it is Schmid who first pointed to Levinas as a hidden resource for person-centred theory. In his 1998 essay on encounter, he puts forward the following criteria for assessing the degree of encounter within therapy. I suggest that these are a sound beginning for assessing person-centred therapy as a spiritual discipline.

---

**Personal Focus 11.2 Peter Schmid's criteria for the quality of encounter and implicitly of spirituality in therapy**

1. Maintain the tension between the sameness and the otherness of the 'We' within the room.
2. Accept the Other in a relationship actually as the Other.
3. In working with the other, put reciprocity into practice.
4. Make the person's capacity for encounter and mutuality an axiom of the relationship.
5. Presence is the existential foundation of the relationship.
6. In being present to the other, be aware of their 'having-become', their historicity.
7. Service is the basic ethic of the relationship from the point of view of the therapist.
8. The psychological includes the physical being and presence of both parties.
9. The group is the basis of all encounter. It offers to all the possibility of meeting and hence of transcendence. Attempt to meet and conceptualize the client as a 'part-of-a-group', as a person-in-relationship.

---

Schmid's criteria are only a beginning, but a very sane beginning, to establish how we might estimate our engagement with the client as spiritual. They are best used by letting them worry you a little. They do not do full justice to all aspects of spirituality, obviously, but they are rooted in the phenomenological and existential perspectives through which spirituality can be more fully explicated. They bring to the fore the question of how spirituality and encounter overlap and interrelate.

# Conclusion

I now refer back to the subtitle of this chapter: phenomenology, existentialism and beyond. The study of the spirituality of counselling, particularly through an awareness of the varied tasks of the discourse, and of the importance of metaphor as a gateway to transcendence, is deeply rooted in the phenomenology and existentialism that is at the heart of person-centred theory and practice. It is phenomenological because it points to the religious and the spiritual as phenomena of human existence. It is existential because it is rooted in values and meaning, in what Sartre (1996) would term the avoidance of bad faith. Yet, it goes beyond the existential to the extent that it insists on the transcendence of human being. In this, it poses the question: What processes in the client and the therapist, and in the space between them, correspond to the transcendent?

If any. Yet, we must decide.

So far in this book, the phenomenological and existential themes have been linked generally to client and therapist process. In the next chapter, the link will be made with the developing thought on person-centred psychopathology, and thence to person-centred practice.

# Further Reading

West, W. (2000) *Psychotherapy and Spirituality*. London, Sage.

This is perhaps a book that all should read. While it is rather too compact and ency-clopaedic, it covers a wide range of theory and practice with a great deal of common sense. William West is a very important contributor in this field. All that he writes should be taken seriously.

Moore, J. and Purton, C. (eds.) (2006) *Spirituality and Counselling: Experiential and Theoretical Perspectives*. Ross-on-Wye, PCCS Books.

A collection of papers from the University of East Anglia 2004 conference 'The Spiritual Dimension in Therapy and Experiential Exploration', this contains many useful papers. However, it also demonstrates as a whole the state of debate on spirituality and counselling today: the writers often fail to *meet* each other.

O'Donohue, J. (1997) *Anam Cara: Spiritual Wisdom from the Celtic World*. London, Bantam Press.

This is a superb example of writing in the Celtic tradition which combines deep personal insight with a thorough philosophical grasp of the tradition. It is the best and most widely useable of spiritual wisdom books.

Worsley, R.J. (2008) 'More than Meets the Eye.' *Therapy Today 19:2*, Rugby, BACP, pp. 34–6.

This is a brief and consumable attempt to make bridges between spirituality and the discipline of group therapy. It attempts a preliminary definition of spirituality from the therapeutic context.

# Part IV
## Moving into Process Work

# 12

# Process in High Levels of Distress: Insights for Everyday Work

The term 'psychopathology' refers to the understanding of patterns of deep distress which cause people to become dysfunctional in a way that inhibits their very living and their level of contact with everyday reality. In books used in initial, person-centred counsellor training in the United Kingdom, it first appeared in the final five chapters of Mearns' (1994b) *Developing Person-Centred Counselling*. In the latest edition of Mearns and Thorne's *Person-Centred Counselling in Action* (2007), this area is given about a third of the chapter on new developments in theory. Psychopathology is an increasingly important area of person-centred theory.

But why does it appear in a book on process work?

1. As person-centred practitioners strive to get their approach taken seriously as psychotherapy, and not just as counselling for the worried-well, we need to take on board the importance of understanding psychopathology. Practising counsellors have increasingly to be in close professional contact with medics and especially psychiatrists and clinical psychologists (Sommerbeck, 2005). While the person-centred model of psychopathology differs radically from the medical model, we must learn both to communicate with the medical profession and to advocate our model and work.
2. The person-centred model of psychopathology is based upon a close understanding of the processes by which clients deal with reality. It is about engaging appropriately with client process, and so is a major element within the territory of this book.
3. I want to put forward the theory that those very processes that mark out psychopathologies which seem on the surface to be difficult, even bizarre, are also to be found in normal range clients, not to mention normal-range therapists. The challenge is this. The more you grasp the processes

behind psychopathological conditions, however exotic they may seem at first glance, the more you will recognize these in 'dilute' forms in your everyday counselling work.

# Precursors to Modern, Person-Centred Psychopathology

At the heart of the person-centred view of psychopathology is the insistence that human distress cannot be likened to a physical illness (Bentall, 2003; Sanders, 2005). Rather it is always expressed as human process, and as such is in tune with Carl Rogers' process formulation of therapy (Rogers, 1957c. See Chapter 3, above). I am finally unwilling to preclude absolutely the presence of biochemical and genetic components to some distress. Yet, claims made by the medical model that it is mainly genetic or a matter of brain chemistry hold little water, as we shall briefly see below. Human distress is multi-factorial – there are many components to it. Physical make-up *may* increase susceptibility but even if it does, that is just one factor. To see distress as process is to accord to it meaning. Being labelled with an illness deprives the experience of meaning. (For a fuller exploration of the relationship of psychiatric diagnosis and labelling to meaning, see my case study of Emma in Worsley, 2007b.)

Why does the person-centred tradition give such emphasis to process with regard to what others often describe as mental illnesses? The answer for me and I guess many practitioners is more to do with experience than theory in itself. As I have come across those who are very distressed, some to the point of being psychotic – having let go of a normal contact with reality – I have been struck that unlike sufferers with influenza, or even those with an organic brain disease like a tumour, the psychotic person seems to be involved in a partially unsuccessful attempt to communicate or even experience their own experiencing.[1] Mearns and Thorne (2007, pp. 32–3) put the matter eloquently:

> We see the results of the actualising process seeking to cope with challenging developmental circumstances and making the best job it can of helping the person to survive and also to develop (albeit within tight limits).

---

[1] Before this, however, a note on language is helpful. It is usual to refer to 'people with autism' rather than 'the autistic', to minimize the effects of labelling. However, there is a real problem with this in term of mental health, and in particular schizophrenia. We will see below that the concept of schizophrenia is highly contestable. To talk of schizophrenia may be a major category error. Therefore I am reluctant to talk of 'people with schizophrenia' as well. I sometimes talk of 'schizophrenics'. By this, I mean those who are so labelled. Perhaps being so labelled socially is the one coherent feature of this so-called group of people! Paradoxically, I am dubious about the more usual turn of phrase because it gives too much credence to the very existence of schizophrenia (Read, 2004).

In other words, the organism attempts to cope in the face of adversity, but sometimes the scale of adversity is such that the coping attempts are themselves highly chaotic. Yet, at some level they work. As with everyday depression, for example, psychosis can be described as a manifestation of incongruence. In Box 12.1, Biermann-Ratjen's (1998, p. 127) description of four typical types of incongruence are set out.

---

### Box 12.1   Four types of incongruence

1. The person may be unable to symbolize completely and communicate verbally certain experiences.
2. The person may be unable to understand and/or accept certain experiences as self- experiences.
3. The person may experience certain ways of defending against experience (stress reactions, acute incongruence) or different forms of stagnation in self-development (chronic incongruence).
4. In any case experiencing incongruence will include experiencing physical tension.

---

Biermann-Ratjen's description of psychotic phenomena in terms of incongruence is informative for a number of reasons. First, it avoids the so-called 'myth of specificity, that each 'mental illness' has a characteristic cause and hence intervention. Rather, the therapist needs to learn from even the most dysfunctional client what meanings and processes are being wrestled with. Secondly, it stresses the connection between familiar person-centred theory and new thinking on psychopathology. Thirdly, its emphasis on the parallels between normal range and psychotic dysfunction in terms of types of incongruence goes some way to explain why we might expect to recognize in normal-range clients some processes that are manifest in psychosis.

Very serious distress is a matter of process and is not at all analogous to physical illness. This radical view is historically rooted in the thought of a number of theorists both within and beyond the person-centred community. These are perhaps the key four:

1. *Gregory Bateson* although born in England worked for much of his life in the United States, and for part of that time he worked in psychiatric hospitals. He was one of the last great polymaths, with expertise in biology, psychology and philosophy. His 1973 book, *Steps towards an Ecology of Mind,* incorporating material from the mid-1950s onwards, strove to establish mindedness as the product of its socio-cultural as well as its biological context.

In so doing, he developed from his work with schizophrenics a learning theory of the condition – specifically the double bind. A double bind is any situation in which it is impossible to win, and this provides a form of mental torment. He came to believe that psychosis was a reaction to the impossibility of demands. It is therefore rooted not in mere biology – and Bateson was a great biologist and geneticist – but in the meaning inherent in torment. While most of us survive intact minor double binds, the great and developmentally significant binds, or the repeated, environmentally saturating ones, generate a deep confusion at the level of the symbolization of experience. The person becomes radically incapable of contextualizing perception and communication. There is poverty of meta-communication. (See Chapter 7 above and Rennie, 1998, chapter eight.)

He tells the story (Bateson, 1973, p. 171) of a young man who had previously lived with his mother, who was a very frightened person, and who expressed this in extreme and obsessive tidiness. The son's double bind was that he was loved but could not live in case he messed things up. Bateson, desperate to communicate with mother, took her some gladioli 'because they are both beautiful and untidy'. She replied, 'Those are not untidy flowers. As each one withers you can snip it off.' And so she had done with her children.

2. *R.D. Laing* was the most celebrated if eccentric of the radical psychiatrists working in the United Kingdom in the middle decades of the twentieth century. He offered in a nutshell a critique of the medical model definition of schizophrenia, which has neither been contradicted by research nor surpassed for cutting brevity:

> There are no pathological anatomical findings *post mortem*. There are no organic structural changes noted in the course of the 'illness'. There are no physiological-pathological changes that can be correlated with these illnesses. There is no general acceptance that any form of treatment is of proven value, except perhaps sustained, careful interpersonal relations and tranquillization. 'Schizophrenia' runs in families, but observes no genetically clear law. It appears usually to have no adverse effect on physical health. [...] It is highly likely that relatively enduring biochemical changes may be the consequence of relatively enduring interpersonal situations of particular kinds.
>
> (Laing and Esterson, 1990, pp. 17–18)

Laing's research established at least at a qualitative level the correlation between unbearable family situations and one member of the family presenting as psychotic. His personal response to this was to set up a therapeutic house in East London. His most famous patient there was Mary Barnes. She wrote up her experience as a book which was then dramatized by David Edgar. Laing demonstrates the link between psychosis and environment, as did Bateson between environment, dysfunction and learning.

3. *John Shlien* was an early pupil of Carl Rogers at the University of Chicago. As early as 1961, he recognized that the person-centred approach offered the potential to work with psychosis, and published a paper putting forward a very preliminary view of schizophrenia (Shlien, 2003, pp. 30–59). His genius is above all in grasping the possibility so early. He describes schizophrenia with reference to Jean-Paul Sartre's notion of 'bad faith' (*la mauvaise foi*). There is colossal incongruence in being itself – an existential failure to take personal responsibility. The 'illness' is then describable in terms of the self-concept. The self-concept in the psychotic person is disorganized and ill-defended, compared with that of the neurotic or paranoid client. There then comes the psychotic break when all that has been denied to awareness overwhelms the self's organization. After this acute phase, patterns of disruption, self-protection and disorganization alternate. The aim of therapy is consequently to help the client re-integrate what is real in experience into a newly organized self-concept.

While Shlien's description of psychosis is not as sophisticated as what was to follow him his key contribution was to link psychosis to the function and process of organismic evaluation of the self.

4. *The Wisconsin Project* stems from Rogers' move to the University of Wisconsin in 1958 (Barrett-Lennard, 1998, pp. 267–73). The project consisted of what might be regarded as two separate sorts of activity. The first was a move on the part of Rogers and others to engage therapeutically with acute and chronic phase schizophrenic, hospitalized patients. The second was a complex exploration of the perceived and rated significance of the relational element in this engagement. The second did not go well. There were elements of mis-design, and elements of misfortune in this failure. However, what emerged was evidence that relational therapy led to recovery and rehabilitation. Rogers' work with Jim over 166 sessions is well-documented as evidence of this (Farber *et al.*, 1996, chapter seven).

In summary, radical psychiatrists and psychologists had brought into question the medical model approach to psychosis. However, those working within the person-centred community had had only a modicum of success in demonstrating the ability of the approach to engage with this group of people. The next stage of development is rich and complex. It is not the task of this chapter to give a full account of this. Rather, the work of Garry Prouty and of Margaret Warner will serve is brief examples for a link to everyday practice.

Before that, I want to point briefly to the critical psychology and psychiatry communities – Bentall (2003), Read *et al.* (2004) and Moncrieff (2008). It is a mistake to ignore our allies in the conceptualization of human distress, just because they do not emerge from our own school of thought.

# Critical Psychology and Psychiatry

As counsellors and psychotherapists, we need our colleagues in critical and positive psychology and psychiatry to save us from the vice of being as simplistic and dogmatic from a person-centred base as are those who with scant regard for good science uphold the dogma of the medical model (Bentall, 2003; Moncrieff, 2008). The very act of summarizing complex material for this chapter has left me feeling nervous in case I sound dogmatic in my own stance. I do not intend to do so. The aim of this section is to outline the key reasons why psychosis should be seen mainly as about meaning and process.

I looked recently at a website – schizophrenia.com – and found it well-meaning but rigidly stuck to the medical model. Its stance was basically that it is comforting to know that schizophrenia is a real illness just like any other and can be cured just like any other. On my way through, I read the following:

> Approximately 40% of people with schizophrenia are unable to understand that they have the disorder, because the part of the brain that is damaged by schizophrenia is also responsible for self-analysis. It's important to note that the person is not 'in denial' (which suggests that through education alone the person might understand that they have schizophrenia). With schizophrenia, you are frequently asking the sick brain to diagnose itself, which may simply be impossible.

What is wrong with this? The answer casts some light upon the short-comings of the medical model. Let us take the statement point by point:

1. If 40 per cent of people with schizophrenia cannot understand they are 'ill', it is very unlikely this is because of brain-damage as part of the disease. Why? Well, there is no explanation as to why 60 per cent can understand. Is it really that something called schizophrenia provides selective brain-damage. Which 40 per cent and why? Evidence? See R.D. Laing above. It makes far more sense to describe this fact in functional – that is, process – terms, the global loss of cognitive insight on a complex continuum.
2. There is part of the brain responsible for self-analysis. This is back-formation from the notion that schizophrenia damages the brain. In fact the neo-cortex is highly complex, and operates by what Edelman (1992) has called very large-scale re-entrant mapping. The brain is highly plastic. Self-analysis is a generalized function of the whole neo-cortex.
3. Schizophrenia damages the brain. But only 40 per cent of schizophrenics in this way! Evidence? More seriously, schizophrenia is not a thing, but a conglomeration of symptoms. It does not damage. That is personification, rhetoric that seduces.
4. 'You are asking the sick brain to diagnose itself.' Note the transition from personal mind language to brain language. I am me, but you are a brain trying to diagnose itself.

5. The underlying motivation of the rhetoric is: Do not worry. It is just another illness. The frustrating bits of schizophrenia are logical enough but without reference to human meaning!
6. Where meaning is reduced, possible guilt on the part of individuals, families and society is minimized (Worsley, 2007b). Medical model thinking has payoffs for clients, families, psychiatrists and drugs firms. It does not mean that this makes it accurate.

We can see that in this one well-meaning paragraph the rhetoric of pseudo-science is seductive. Critical psychology and psychiatry invites us to question the basis in logic, philosophy, science and research of mental health orthodoxy. What follows are brief examples of this.

*Soteria* was a project in the United States. It ran from 1961 until closed through the withdrawal of funding in 1983. It was a lay community of helpers and of schizophrenic people who were mainly drug-free. It demonstrated that the key qualities of healing in psychosis are about community and relationship. This experience was twice repeated in Europe. It demonstrated that human relating is a crucial corrective in psychosis and that the main advantage to working with first episode clients without drugs was that the appalling side-effects of psycho-active drugs were avoided (Read *et al.*, 2004, chapter 24; Moncrieff, 2008, *passim*).

*Joanna Moncrieff* is an academic and clinical psychiatrist who teaches at University College, London. The bulk of her research profile concerns itself with analysis of the effects and effectiveness of the drugs used in the treatment of mental health conditions. Her recent book (Moncrieff, 2008) gives a detailed account of the evidential base for the effectiveness of many psychiatric drugs. She concludes that they are in general little more effective than the placebo effect, but carry varying levels of severe and damaging side-effects. Perhaps her most powerful argument is that psychoactive drugs are strongly sedative or stimulant, and that this can be of some use, just as alcohol helps with confidence. But it does not 'cure' a 'disease'. She concludes and demonstrates that their use is not unrelated to the marketing efforts of the drug companies. For Moncrieff, the chemical cure is a myth generated for profit as well as out of a misapplication of the medical model.

*Richard Bentall* is Professor of Experimental Clinical Psychology at the University of Manchester. His 2003 book is a comprehensive analysis of psychosis and its various treatments. His deconstruction of schizophrenia in particular – supported by the work of his New Zealand colleague, John Read (2004) – is thorough and expert. His key points are the following:

1. There is no definitive line between normality and madness.
2. Schizophrenia is not a coherent idea, because the vast majority of schizophrenics do not share the majority of symptoms. It is like saying that some who suffer from influenza have red spots and no congestion, while

the rest have congestion but no spots, yet it is all influenza! Technically speaking, the concept has low validity.

3. Specifically, the symptoms of the condition seem to fall into three groups, which are better regarded as three different complexes of conditions rather than a single disease.
4. Thirty years after Laing made the point, there is still no biological or physiological component common to all schizophrenics.
5. Diagnoses are notoriously imprecise, when one clinician's judgement is compared with another's. The concept of schizophrenia has what is technically known as low reliability.
6. The medical model prevents the addressing of the patient's psychological needs.

Sanders (2005, p. 29) sums up the findings thus:

So a significant group of critical psychologists, academics and psychiatrists have discovered that the best way to help chronically distressed people is to offer them:

1. Relationships...
2. that are characterized by interpersonal, phenomenologic interventions,
3. offered by non-professional staff (not medically qualified),
4. who relate to the client as a person, not a distant and powerful expert,
5. where the staff help clients understand implicit meaning in their experiences and
6. value clients' experiences, treating them with respect
7. in growth-oriented, supportive communities, not hospital/medical settings.

## Contact

> If you need to give and receive *too much* 'love', you will be at high risk of diagnosis from schizophrenia. The diagnosis attributes to you the incapacity, by and large, to give or receive 'love' in an adult manner. When you smile at such a thought, this may confirm the diagnosis since you are suffering from 'inappropriate affect'.
>
> (Laing, 1961, p. 107)

Gregory Bateson and R.D. Laing, *inter alii*, had shown that schizophrenia was more to do with meaning than genetics. Richard Bentall and John Read have subsequently demonstrated the unreliability and invalidity of schizophrenia as a coherent disease. Laing and Loren Mosher, on opposite sides of the Atlantic, have demonstrated the power of community as a healing power, and therefore again of meaning and socio-psychological context as key factors (Sanders,

2007a). Diagnosis is therefore an imprecise art form to put it mildly. Whatever the shortcomings of the Wisconsin project, Rogers, like Shlien, had shown case evidence of the impact of person-centred therapy upon people diagnosed with schizophrenia. Yet, if the whole concept of schizophrenia is contestible, there was yet to be revealed a common factor for all psychoses.

In 1966, a pupil of Eugene Gendlin (see Chapter 2) began work with a group of clients who were both diagnosed as schizophrenic and who had learning disabilities too. This was Garry Prouty. At first he believed that he was working in a classically client-centred way with the clients, but after looking in detail at his interventions with some of his students, he was persuaded that he had inadvertently alighted upon a new way of communicating (Prouty *et al.*, 2002, pp. 7–8). From this analysis he developed his theory and practice of pre-therapy. The principle of it is simplicity itself.

Rogers' (1957a, 1959) papers stating the six conditions of therapy had begun with the fact that the therapist and the client need to be in psychological contact. He defines this as each making a minimal impact upon the other's phenomenal field. While it is often said that psychotic people are out of touch with reality, this truth has a more precise form. In florid psychosis, there is no contact. Rogers had worked, for example with Jim Brown in 1962 (Farber *et al.*, 1996, pp. 231–60). Jim had been so wounded by those close to him that he had retreated into silence, cut off from all others. After some 160 hours of therapy, Rogers in sticking with Jim in his profound silence, his being cut off, rebuilt contact in the technical sense, as well as human trust. Prouty's major insight – as much from his personal experience as his clinical and philosophical knowledge – was that contact requires a grounding in the concrete. This is true for us all; it is merely that we take it for granted. In psychosis, this grounding in the concrete is lost and awaits recovery. Therefore, Prouty realized that what he had been doing with his very distressed client group was to reflect back concrete facts very literally. However, it is worth noting before we move into practice issues that the continuum between normal and psychotic experience is evident to us all, as Personal Focus 12.1 indicates:

---

**Personal Focus 12.1   Normally psychotic**

Six days ago, a close friend died in difficult circumstances. I feel grief and anger, but I am not sure where to place the anger. God? The hospital? Life?

Last night, after four hours of sleep, I awoke. I am not aware that I was dreaming. (Maybe it would have been better if I had dreamt.) As I lay in bed, I realized that I felt not just restless or in need of some water, but rather that I felt disturbed. I actually struggle to describe how I felt. Perhaps that is the point. It did not fit easily into words.

I felt deeply depressed, rather than sad. I can only describe it as a crumbling of something that I cannot identify. In a short period of time, I had processed a number of resentments and fears. There was the schoolboy by whom I felt bullied; and the friend from long ago who had betrayed me politically. There was a sense of my faith falling apart. At the same time I was terrified that I would have to resign my job as a counsellor because I must be becoming dysfunctional. At the age of 56, I felt scared and *very* old. What I can't describe is how the whole of this came together as a world that I hated and could not cope with. It was symbolized for me by the sense of detestation I suddenly felt for Robert Mugabe. All in the space of a few minutes I knew I lived on a blighted planet that was cursed with both a food shortage and climate disaster. I really did not want to live. Why could I not have died like my parents when the world was happy?

My wife, who had by then awoken as well, asked me what was wrong. If I am a bit down or worried, I will often not want to talk about it. On this occasion, I heard myself say, I am really rather worried about myself, my mental state. I described in only a couple of sentences the feelings that were going through me. She heard what I said but gave me minimal response – I think because she was tired! Within ten minutes, and a cup of tea later, I felt better, I can only say, sane again.

This was not madness, but a sleeping way of processing grief and anger and anxiety. I am struck by the similarity of my own distorted experience to psychotic experience. The exception was that I was able to use my wife's question to ground myself. *When talking recently to a paranoid client I recognized that the main difference between us was that he took three days rather than ten minutes to process his paranoid thinking.*

Can you locate experiences like this of 'sane psychosis'?

I hope that the feel of Personal Focus 12.1 is clear to the reader – that psychotic-type processing is part of normal life, under stress. This was first observed by Sigmund Freud, that psychotic thinking much resembles dreaming. He termed this 'primary process'.

## Theory and Practice – Pre-therapy

Garry Prouty began to discover the potentiality of pre-therapy from 1966 on (Prouty *et al.*, 2002, pp. 3–6). The essential realization on his part was that psychosis and severe learning needs both involved a lack of contact between the person and her environment. On reviewing the way he found himself working with such clients, he came to recognize, and then to theorize, the need to make concrete his reflections and empathy. A persistent and reliable reflection of the concrete is at the heart of his practice. In Box 12.2, I list his categories of reflection and then the three major guidelines for practice which undergird these (Prouty *et al.*, 2002, pp. 11–13, 16):

---

### Box 12.2 Prouty's reflections

*Situational Reflection*: The therapist reflects the client's behaviour in relation to her situation or environment.

*Facial Reflection*: The therapist looks at the client's face and reflects her expressive affect, such as 'Leanne looks angry'.

*Body Reflection*: Reflecting body posture, which can help the client overcome her alienation from her own body.

*Word-for-word Reflections*: Empathic yet very literal reflection of what the client said. Psychotic clients appear to struggle to understand paraphrasing (Warner, 2007).

*Re-iterative Reflections*: A return to a previous point of contact, which may be two minutes ago, of maybe last week. 'Last week you said "baby". Now you hold a doll.'

**Three Principles:**

1. Respond to the direct experience of what is there.
2. Respond to the client's naturalistic and realistic sense when it is there.
3. Look as much as you listen.

---

You will notice that these responses are very literal. At first, they feel awkward, mechanical. The aim is to be in empathic attitude in spite of this initial feeling. In practice, the most obvious use of such reflections is with those who are lapsing into psychotic episode.

---

### Case 12.1 Coping in a crisis

Arlene was referred to me by a personal tutor, because she was anxious about what she was dealing with. I managed to see her straight away. It was the first week of term. She told me, hesitantly, that she had been home for the vacation, but had been pursued by a stalker.

At first, the story made quite a bit of sense, but over a period of some 15 minutes, it felt less real, more delusional. I asked Arlen where the stalker was now. She replied that he had followed her to University. This seemed unlikely. I needed to get her to the Health Centre for assessment. She was very frightened and very reluctant to agree, but did so when I said I would go with her. I left her in my room for a few minutes to make the relevant phone call, and to touch base with a colleague too. When I returned to my room, she looked at me, still terrified, and said, 'You are not the same man!'

I felt simultaneously a great relief that this confirmed my anxiety that Arlene was lapsing fast into psychotic episode and a thrownness as to how to reply. I looked at her as calmly as I could – I think striving to reassure us both – and said. 'I left the room to make a phone call. (*Situational Reflection*) When I come back, you look scared (*Facial Reflection*) and you say to me: You are not the same man! (*Word-for-word Reflection*.)'

Arlene became calmer, and was able to accompany me to the Health Centre and wait with me until I could hand her over to a G.P. In a situation of much fear, I had managed to give her enough that is concrete to ground her.

At its simplest, pre-therapy looks to be almost bizarrely straightforward. However, Prouty has theorized these procedures with some sophistication. In psychosis, there is a break in the client's contact with reality. Prouty sees this as a structural deficit in experience. Experience refers only to itself and not beyond itself. Therefore it has meaning, but the grammar of this meaning is not the same as in normal functioning (Prouty *et al.*, 2002, chapters 2 and 5; Prouty, 2007). Prouty sees pre-therapy as that which regains contact and makes possible therapy. By contrast, Van Werde (2002, 2005, 2007) sees pre-therapy as in and of itself therapeutic, particularly when its theory and practice are integrated into the milieu of a residential setting.

Case 12.1 is an example of the practical usefulness of Prouty's procedures. Yet, both pre-therapy and other existential understandings of psychosis give us access to processes which also exist, in varying degrees, in normal-range functioning. To consider this further, we move on to the work of the American academic and clinician, Margaret Warner.

## Theory and Practice – Metaphact and Metacause

A nurse was engaged to look after a somewhat catatonic, hebephrenic, schizophrenic patient. Shortly after they met, the nurse gave the patient a cup of tea. The chronically psychotic patient, on taking the tea, said, 'This is the first time in my life that anyone has ever given me a cup of tea'.

(Laing, 1961, p. 106)

Rogers (1957c) made it clear that one of the processes which make for healthy, which is to say congruent, living is our ability to symbolize, to express and to make explicit when necessary our experiencing both to ourselves and to others. Eugene Gendlin (1981, 1997) elaborated upon this by describing the way that meaning, far from being a set of merely cognitive beliefs, is something which is first of all *felt*. He hypothesizes that meaning and emotion emerge from within as a bodily felt-sense, and only then, and at times gradually, do they become fully conscious and formulated. Metaphors (see Chapter 5) are particularly important in this process in that they can express felt-sense and felt-meaning through pictures. However, it is not merely pictures as illustrations or linguistic decoration. Metaphors can embody the process of symbolizing our meanings. There is always a surplus of meaning to be had from metaphor. What a metaphor 'contains', how I use it to allow my meaning and emotion to emerge for me is without limit, infinite (Ricoeur, 1975).

Metaphor is therefore of key importance in working with psychosis. Psychosis might be seen as meaning that cannot emerge – for whatever reason. Metaphor in psychosis moves away from the normal function of imaginative and generative process, which allows meaning to emerge as felt and then fully symbolized. Rather metaphor becomes a desperate struggle to communicate across a chasm of isolation and fear. The dynamics of communication change.

In the vignette from Laing (1961) at the head of this section, the psychotic young man says that it is the first time that anyone has given him a cup of tea. This is, of course, like madness. Laing comments later that the patient's life-experience suggests that the image he creates is almost literally true. Had he said to the nurse, 'The way you look after me is something I've never experienced before!' then we would have understood. But the experience as felt is translated into a statement that sounds unlikely. Is it literally the case? If not, the patient is constructing a metaphor that both does and does not communicate. We might reasonably ask what in this young man's life makes it so unrewarding or so dangerous to seek to get his needs met, that the *cri de coeur* must be so loud and so hidden. He is catatonic and hebephrenic. That is to say, he usually stands paralysed and, when he does communicate, does so in a juvenile way. The metaphor here is remarkable for its congruence. It also says, 'You have won my trust enough for me to say what I need, but I still dare not come quite straight out with it.'

Look back again to Personal Focus 12.1. It may not have been obvious why I saw my state of mind at 4am as paralleling that of psychosis. I had got everything out of proportion. The literal stress was the grief I felt at the death of my friend and the underlying existential impact of it as a reminder of my own mortality. While in the cool light of morning I can reflect on that, the raw fact of it on the borders of sleep was unbearable. It was as if reality was threatened. Each anxiety and threat to self, others and the world, from the crumbling of my world-view through my memory of being bullied to my concern for the people of Zimbabwe, all these became metaphors, one for another and all together for the anxiety provoked by loss. I was in the midst of a miniature madness. I am loath to see this as 'loss of reality', but perhaps more the true force of reality. I could ground myself. In Prouty's terms, the images of mortality ceased to be self-referential and hence unconnected, and became processed as fully symbolic. The psychotic person may take days to find this grounding, or it may be absent for months. Yet, my experience-in-miniature suggests to me that madness is closer to reality in some (metaphorical?) senses than would be sanity.

I now move on to Margaret Warner's (2007) case study of Luke. Luke shows elements of schizophrenic thought disorder. Warner has worked with him for some 13 years, at the date of writing. Warner is, for me, exceptional in that she derives so much insight from case work. Too often, mental health issues are classified according to medical model theory rather than through learning to listen to the client (Moncrieff, 2008). Warner had felt fear of Luke in the early days – or perhaps fear of her own lack of competence. She learned to listen to him, and realized that two things were true. When she paraphrased Luke, in a way that one would with a normal-range client, he was often unable to understand what she was saying, and became very scared of this failure to understand. However, when she stuck fairly precisely to Luke's words, he felt understood, but, more to the point, Warner came to grasp more and more of Luke's world, even when she did not fully grasp the sense of what she was reflecting. Her intention here is different from Prouty's: for Prouty, the intention is to root the client in the concreteness of experience, while for Warner it is merely to avoid confusing Luke by varying his language. She had come to experience the communicational nature of Luke's thought disorder. But in what way was Luke thinking or speaking differently? (Thought and speech are perhaps not too separate.)

Her clue came in listening to Luke's inability to deal with metaphors:

> One day Luke had lunch with his father and a Catholic priest who was a family friend. The priest lamented the fact that in recent days Catholics were 'going to the dogs'. Luke, who is Catholic, had never considered the possibility that he might be about to become a dog. But, he spent the next weekend carefully scrutinizing dogs he saw in the park to see how they were doing. He decided that they mostly seemed to have smiles on their faces, so, he came to the conclusion that turning into a dog might not be such a terrible thing.
>
> (Warner, 2007, p. 142)

Imagine only how much more difficult this would be if it *was* awful to Luke to become a dog. The torment would be horrific. Warner developed from this and other examples her notion of metaphact and its parallel concept, the metacause. A metaphact is an idea that combines aspects of fact and metaphor with an inability to make clear distinctions between the two. The metacause is a similar failure to grasp causal chains and associations which normal-range people largely can take for granted.

Warner combined her discipline of remaining as close as possible to Luke's words and thinking hard about the nature of the metaphact. For example, Luke commented on one occasion that his father could scarcely understand him, because he was Spanish and came from a different country. However, Luke noted, he could understand his father so they must come from the same country. We can notice two things about this. The first is that if Luke had used the language of metaphor normally by saying that it was *as if* his father experienced him speaking another language, this would have been an unexceptional statement. The second is that the metacausal property of this communication by Luke is that the *same country/different country* contradiction does not matter. (Freud had observed that primary process contains no contradictions. We do not object to a dream because it includes patent nonsense!) By tolerating the quality of the communication in terms of metaphact and metacause, Warner was able to empathize with the existential experience of Luke, that his father did not understand him.

Warner's approach is then to remain close to Luke's words, to try to be aware of the nature of what he wants to communicate, and not to try to teach him to work normally. (I hypothesize that the last of these is truer for dysfunctional psychotic processing than it is for more functional processing – perhaps by definition. I could reprocess my quasi-psychotic process after sleep in part by 'learning' that I had done it wrong.) She summarizes the outcome for Luke thus:

> In my observation of Luke, he seems to have made a great deal of progress in finding ways to process effectively using metaphact language. His process is slower than a more normative client's process might be since he needs to make sense of many aspects of situations that would be processed quasi-automatically by most people. (For example, a server in the coffee shop who smiles at him can be quite puzzling to him.) And, given the difficulty forming clear units and causes in metaphact language, Luke sometimes has trouble making sense of particular logical aspects of personal situations. (For example he has difficulty understanding why people would think that smoking cigarettes would give a person cancer.) But, in spite of these limitations, metaphact process is very effective in clarifying Luke's understandings of what is bothering him, why it bothers him and what he would like to have happen.
>
> (Warner, 2007, p. 150)

How can this inform work with clients who are less disordered than Luke. For the purpose, I want to return to the case of Angélique, who we met in Chapter 5. There I had considered my work with her in terms of her configurations and her ability to contain her paranoid self within one configuration. (This construct may correspond closely to Garry Prouty's (2007) hypothesis that in psychotic experience the hallucination represents the dissociated or unsymbolized part of the client.) Here, I want to think about the way I tried to facilitate this containment:

---

### Case 12.2  Angélique Reconsidered

*Please refer back to Chapter 5 and page 85 for details in the case of Angélique.*

Angélique experienced paranoid thinking especially at work. It is a feasible interpretation of this to see work as the place where the paradoxical threat, the double bind, was strongest. If she failed she betrayed her father's script for her; if she succeeded, she was 'unfeminine' on the surface, but underneath in the unspoken territory of her mother's anxiety – responsibility beyond the tolerable.

Angélique's paranoia was clearly problematical. At best she felt uncertain as to whether this situation or that were a threat and at worst she became convinced that others were trying to harm her. I begin by noting that there are many real-life situations in which the uncertainty is both normal and necessary.

A woman walks home along a dark lane. She is alone at first. There are no people or houses in easy reach. Before she gets to her village, she becomes aware of a man (Is it a man? Another woman?) following her. She quickens her pace. Is she in danger? It would be disproportionate to be certain that she was. Yet, it would be foolish to presume she was not. Fear of attack preserves life.

We are prone to label Angélique as non-normal because her fear of others seems unjustified – to me, that is! The paranoia is clear enough, it seems. But perhaps the more important question is what makes Angélique normal. Although having moments of intense stress and irrational certainty, she is able to hold an internal discussion with herself about that notion of some of her thinking being paranoid. She can entertain within herself a number of possible versions of the truth. She can process these. The difference between her and the woman in the dark lane is that she has to work harder and more slowly to strike some sense of balance. The way things are fluctuate for Angélique.

Yet, her normality, if you like, is grounded in her self-contact. She can symbolize to herself her range of experiences (Rogers, 1957c), including a meta-experience of comparing different levels of fear at different times. It is from this symbolization that she can negotiate who she is. I take it to be the case that the psychotic break, the point at which this ability to reflect critically upon experience, is lost is at the point of loss of contact with the self and with the outside world. This observation is particularly in tune with van Werde's (2002, 2005) argument that pre-therapy type contact work need only from 20 to 30 per cent of the work of his ward for the therapeutic effect of all work to be greatly enhanced.

What then are the practice implications for this conceptualization of Angélique?

1. At first I listened with empathy to a woman who was obviously deeply distressed. This was not too difficult, until it began to occur to me that I simply did not believe all that she was telling me. The word paranoid came to me.

2. It would be very tempting to back away at that point. The disorientated perceptions of the mad parts of us need as much accompaniment and understanding – perhaps even more – than our saner selves. Remain genuinely empathic to the experience.

3. Listen also for that part of the client that may be able to access a different perspective. If that part is not available, there is a question of practitioner competence. Should you be working with this client? Is the client available enough for therapy? Is pre-therapy something that you can practice? Training? Would other sorts of psychiatric support be useful? (Remember that Moncrieff, 2008, argues that drugs are useful, as long as their use is conceived of in a drug-centred scheme.)

4. Monitoring the above as you proceed continue to remain in touch with the feelings which underlie the metaphacts of the hallucination.

5. Be cautious not to offer an interpretation (your truth and that of 'professionals'). Can the client develop a conversation between the reflective and the non-reflective parts of her self?

6. Be prepared to be flexible about psycho-education. Does it help to explain to the client how she might think about her experience? It did help Angélique to see that her paranoia, which she knew well enough, could be linked to her experience of how she had grown up with mother. The same was not true for Margaret Warner in her work with Luke. She thinks of being asked,

**Couldn't you just explain to Luke that he is blurring facts and metaphors and teach him to think in more normative ways?** I've never tried this, but I don't think that it would work. I've heard Luke describe innumerable interactions in which Sheffield House staff or family members try to explain emotionally-loaded subjects (like why he shouldn't smoke) with normative cause-effect logics. Luke feels quite confused by these explanations. He takes in the explanations through the same metaphact lens with which he takes in other novel information, blurring facts and metaphors. Often, rather than making things clear to him, these explanations lead him to give up on understanding what is going on. Instead, he just tries to fake it, trying to meet other people's expectations. Or, he stubbornly refuses to go along while not being willing to explain why.

(Warner, 2007, p. 154)

7. See the work as helping the client to symbolize her own experience, both the paranoid and the normal, and to thence become a manager of her varied experience. Do not discriminate against the psychotic. It is valuable. It embodies that which cannot/has not yet been symbolized.

This chapter has asked what can be learned about the process of all clients from the so-called 'psychopathological'. The result is a number of insights, but not a coherent model of process. In the next chapter, a case study of Hilary will be matched against one consistent model of process, as set out in Greenberg *et al.* (1993).

# Further Reading

## *General*

Sanders, P. (ed.) (2007b) *The Contact Work Primer: A concise, accessible and comprehensive introduction to Pre-Therapy and the work of Garry Prouty*. Ross-on-Wye, PCCS Books.

　　The best short introduction to the whole area of concern.

Joseph, S. and R.J. Worsley (eds.) (2005) *Person-Centred Psychopathology: A positive psychology of mental health*. Ross-on-Wye, PCCS Books.
Worsley, R.J. and S. Joseph (eds.) (2007) Person-*Centred Practice: Case studies in positive psychology*. Ross-on-Wye, PCCS Books.

　　Two recent and important collections of essays from international, person-centred scholars, the first is about theory and the second is a series of case studies. They are perhaps the best general introduction to the field at the moment. The logical starting point is with Pete Sanders' critique of the medical model, being chapter three of Joseph and Worsley (2005).

Prouty, G.F., Van Werde, D. and Pörtner, M. (2002) *Pre-therapy: Reaching contact-impaired clients*. Ross-on-Wye, PCCS Books.

This is an important introduction to the specific territory of pre-therapy. It is worth noting that Prouty sees pre-therapy as literally that which is prior to any therapy, while Van Werde makes the case for it being itself therapeutic.

## Contact and the Actualizing Tendency

Levitt, B.E. (ed.) (2008) *Reflections on Human Potential: Bridging the Person-Centred Approach and Positive Psychology*. Ross-on-Wye, PCCS Books.
Wyatt, G. and Sanders, P. (eds.) (2002) *Contact and Perception*. Ross-on-Wye, PCCS Books.

Contact and the actualizing tendency are the two key concepts in person-centred theory for the understanding of a person-centred psychopathology. Both of these books are creative meditations upon these themes.

## Critical Psychology and Psychiatry

Bentall, R.P. (2003) *Madness Explained: Psychosis and Human Nature*. Harmondsworth, Penguin.
Moncrieff, J. (2008) *The Myth of the Chemical Cure: A Critique of Psychiatric Drug Treatment*. Houndmills, Palgrave.
Read, J., Mosher, L.R. and Bentall, R. (eds.) (2004) *Models of Madness: Psychological, Social and Biological Approaches to Schizophrenia*. London, Brunner-Routledge.

All four authors of these three texts offer a clear and challenging critique of the medical model of distress, with particular reference to schizophrenia. Bentall and Read are psychologists, Mosher and Moncrieff, psychiatrists. To get to grips with these three books is to begin to develop a sound mode of defending the person-centred approach to psychopathology.

# 13

# A Process Paradigm and Hilary: A Case Study of One Moment of Process Work

## Clients and Models: The Specificity Myth

So far the underlying argument of this book has been simple enough. It puts forward three key points:

1. A client's process is as much an aspect of their frame of reference as are other aspects of their awareness. To understand process is a form of empathy.
2. It is not the case – *pace* Rennie and others – that the client is the expert on her content and the therapist upon her process. Therapists have expertise based upon an experience of the uniqueness of all of their clients. Thus in respect of process, the therapist needs to learn from the client as well, through mutual exploration of the quality of experiencing.
3. Therapists need to use theory – be it that of Rogers or Perls or Berne or whoever – to understand ways of conceptualizing and expressing process. Theory is always a schematization of, and hence approximation to, psychological reality.

The key point throughout is that the therapist learns from each client her unique pattern of processing.

In this chapter I will set out the key theoretical principles of the paradigm of therapy proposed by Les Greenberg, Laura Rice and Robert Elliott (Greenberg *et al.*, 1993) (henceforth, the paradigm). The theory of the paradigm, which has been further elaborated in, for instance, Elliott *et al.*, 2003 describes the complex relationship of thinking and emotions and the variety of patterns (schemata and schemas) by which they interrelate. This description in turn allows us to be more aware of which aspects of our underlying patterns change easily, and which tend to resist change. We will see this awareness in action in the case study of Hilary.

However, beyond this fertile theory, the paradigm describes six therapeutic tasks which correspond to six characteristic modes of dysfunction. Such specificity becomes a vice when it attempts to link 'treatments' to specific categories as though each category would obligingly function like an illness.

In short, the theory of the paradigm is a valuable resource for conceptualizing the client's unique ways of processing. When it slips into diagnosis, many person-centred practitioners would want to dissent from it.

---

### Personal Focus 13.1   Thinking about Diagnosis

My client was a young woman aged 19. She was distressed, panicky, agitated, and at times fairly deeply depressed. She said that she had seen a community psychiatric nurse who had said to her: I think you have bipolar disorder, *but you do not yet fit.*

In the next session, my client told me that six months previously a close friend of her own age had died of a drug overdose. She had been deeply affected but had told no one and had talked to no one about it. It was her first experience of anyone close to her dying. A return to sadness and health came relatively swiftly.

---

## Paradigms

All thinking about theory, in any subject, tends to be paradigmatic. That is to say, we do not think radically new thoughts whenever we try to describe patterns and understandings. We live in communities and societies that pass on to us ways of thinking. We tend to live within these thought-contexts quite conservatively. A paradigm is a template for thinking.

There is a Buddhist story – I cannot remember where I heard or read it – of a person who went to visit a wise monk to learn about living more fully. At first, the monk said nothing of value. As time went on, the visitor became more and more irritated and then outraged. Time was being wasted! In the end, anger drove the visitor to demand the wisdom that she sought. The wise monk replied that he would only reveal wisdom on one condition: 'When you came into my house, you removed your shoes. Tell me how you left them.' The visitor was pole-axed. She had no memory of her shoes.

In this story there are a number of elements. The main point is that wisdom comes from awareness. However, the story might also represent in microcosm the meeting of Eastern and Western thinking. The visitor had expected that wisdom could be told; the monk knew that it had to be lived. The visitor came with one paradigm of wisdom, and had to switch to another. The new paradigm seemed no doubt to her more difficult because less familiar.

Counselling theory works in paradigms too. Each of the major approaches is a paradigm of psychological and therapeutic thinking. One of the key themes of this book has been to expand the thinking and experiencing of person-centred practice so as to affirm contact with the broader resources of the humanistic and existentialist traditions, and in particular to show how person-centred practice can remain true to itself while addressing process. This book advocates a paradigm shift, albeit a fairly conservative one.

As part of this, I want to offer the paradigm as an insight which I have found to be profoundly helpful.

## Introducing the Paradigm

*Facilitating Emotional Change: The Moment-by-Moment Process* (Greenberg *et al.*, 1993) is an important book, but not an easy one to read. It is crucial to understand that the book has two quite separate purposes and that I am interested in and convinced by only the first of these.

The first 95 pages of the book aim to produce a description of the nature of emotional change and thus of what it is, at least in part, to be human. This description strives to unite the insights of Carl Rogers and Fritz Perls. It is debatable whether it succeeds, but for me that is of no consequence. It has a validity of its own. This first section uses the authors' deep knowledge of research and theory in cognitive science and emotion theory to generate a new understanding of the process of emotional change, but an understanding which is in the main coherent with the work of Carl Rogers.

The remainder of this chapter will take main themes from the paradigm and describe them in as practical a fashion as possible, linking them to casework experience.

The paradigm has three major virtues for me:

1. It is largely congruent with Rogers' theory, and in fact helps to resolve some tensions in this around the notion of the actualizing tendency, by setting Rogers' thought in the context of evolutionary theory.

2. It gives a coherent description of the relationship between spontaneity and reflexivity.
3. Above all, it offers an answer on behalf of the depth psychologies to the argument of cognitive therapy that if only the client were to think straight then their feelings would follow. The paradigm offers a rebuttal to those cognitive practitioners who see depth work as inefficient and therefore self-indulgent.

# The Paradigm

Figure 13.1 is a diagram of the paradigm. This is to me, a highly useful illustration and I am grateful to the group of my students who refused to hide their lack of understanding, so that between us we had to draw it.

## *Five Strands of Cognitive Science*

In their review of cognitive science research, Greenberg *et al.* (1993) points to five principles. Each is rooted in empirical study and research. They govern the way that we can think about client (and counsellor) process:

1. In the evolution of the brain and the mind it is clear that attention, and the self-consciousness which flows from our ability to pay attention, is an important human resource. Without this we would be little better than living automata. However, attention has its problems. It is a scarce resource and it needs to be so. If we paid attention in equal amounts to all potential experience we would soon be swamped. In addition, automatic reactions like the reflexes and the fight–flight mechanism have a high value in self-preservation in dangerous environments. Paying attention to one stimulus and therefore not to others requires a level of environmental safety.

   We pay attention only to a very small part of all of our experiencing. We experience patterns (*Gestalten*) only as a result of selecting particular characteristics of objects for attention (Harris, 2003, chapter one). In therapy, we aim to help clients use their attention-giving creatively.
2. Some of our thinking and a large amount of our feeling happens at least in the first instance out of our focused awareness (Gendlin, 1997).
3. The human brain demonstrates two sorts of processing, which have their analogues in computer-processing, even though there are clear and major differences between brains and computers. Serial processing is slow, real-time processing and likely to be in awareness. Parallel processing is very

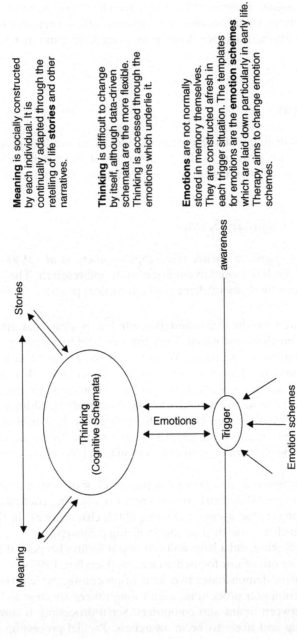

**Meaning** is socially constructed by each individual. It is continually adapted through the retelling of life **stories** and other narratives.

**Thinking** is difficult to change by itself, although data-driven schemata are the more flexible. Thinking is accessed through the emotions which underlie it.

**Emotions** are not normally stored in memory themselves. They are constructed afresh in each trigger situation. The templates for emotions are the **emotion schemes** which are laid down particularly in early life. Therapy aims to change emotion schemes.

Stories

Meaning

Thinking (Cognitive Schemata)

Emotions

Trigger

awareness

Emotion schemes

*Figure 13.1* A diagrammatic representation of the principles behind the theory of cognitive-affective psychology of Greenberg *et al.* (1993) *Facilitating Emotional Change*

fast, has a high self-preservation function in situations of danger, and is mostly out of focused awareness.

---

**Personal Focus 13.2   Selective awareness**

Choose an object to focus your awareness on. Perhaps it is useful if it is an enjoyable object such as a plant or picture. Focus as hard on this object as you can for a few moments. What do you notice about the object? After a short while, maintain your focused awareness, but try to be aware also of your surroundings. What do you notice about the surroundings and the object? About the act of maintaining your focus of awareness?

Recall an instance when you were quite severely startled. What did you experience? What might you understand by the evolutionary significance of this? How would your startle reflex help you in a dangerous situation?

---

4. Memory is dynamic and reconstructive. This means that we do not *store* memories on a large scale, particularly in terms of emotion or emotionally coloured events. Rather, we store schemes and schemata (see below for the difference) which enable us to construct afresh our emotional and even cognitive responses to situations.
5. There are two sorts of templates which we store. Emotion schemes are fundamental patterns of the way we assemble our feeling self at each point in time. Cognitive schemata – patterns of ways of thinking – are often derived from, or are dependent upon, emotion schemes.

Thinking processes are difficult to change in themselves, because thinking and emotion cannot be separated out. Therapy often involves the client accessing the emotion scheme and then the cognitive schema in order to construct new meaning.

---

**Personal Focus 13.3   Spontaneous and reflexive feeling**

Relax and clear your mind. Recall an episode that evoked a strong emotional reaction in you. Let that event come back for you. (I suggest a pleasant rather than a difficult situation.)

Be aware of how you immediately experience that recall. Where in your body does the emotion begin to emerge?

Continue to feel that experience as openly as you can.

- What did it mean to you? Concentrate on its meaning. Try and explain that to an imaginary other person.
- What differences did it make to move from a reflexive approach to an emotional experience? Speed? Detail? Focus of awareness?

## Cognitive Schemata

It is conventional to refer to a cognitive map as a schema (plural, schemata) and to emotion maps as schemes.

The brain does not store information in small, unrelated packages in the way that a computer does in Random Access Memory. The brain stores information and then plans of information at many levels of complexity. Edelman (1992) describes the process of accessing very complex plans as 'large-scale re-entrant mapping'. The brain, in other words, has the ability to consult its own library of schemes and schemata to discover how it needs to feel and think. We do not learn to think each time we do think. That would be hopelessly inefficient. We *learn*.

Our cognitive schemata come in two varieties. Concept-driven schemata are 'top–down'. We think by unconsciously consulting a set of principles that we have already learned and then we apply them. Concept-driven schemata are very resistant to change. It is these which operate when we experience ourselves as being 'stuck in our heads'. However, their very conservatism is of evolutionary advantage. I would never go to work if I had to re-decide my whole political philosophy every time I woke up!

Data-driven schemata are open to consult incoming information (including emotional information) and are thus far more flexible. Rogers (1957c) suggests that being fully functioning involves openness to the world, and thus perhaps involves a move from concept-driven schemata to data-driven schemata. The latter, being more adaptable, will enable the person to be more congruent with the environment.

### Personal Focus 13.4   Changing cognitive schemata

- Contact your religious or political belief system. State for yourself roughly what it contains. What makes me a socialist? An atheist?
- When did you last experience a major change in your belief system? What brought this about? How did it feel?
- Our political and religious affiliations are normally (but not always) concept-driven. 'This is my identity.' They change slowly and reluctantly. Is this true for you?

▪ Recall the last piece of positive feedback that you received. It need not be about a major issue. Let yourself bathe for a few moments in its after-glow.

▪ Even in small ways, did you experience any change in the way you see yourself as a result of that feedback?

▪ Feedback in the more functional person often construes data-driven schemata. These are more flexible. Do you experience changes in yourself and your self-concept when you receive feedback?

---

### Box 13.1  Therapy and cognitive schemata

▪ Your ideas will not tend to change your clients' ideas about themselves. Teaching is far less effective than facilitating learning.

▪ Congruent, empathic and accepting relating involves feedback given and received both in and out of awareness.

▪ As a client feels accepted, so he can accept the therapist's care for him, even when the feedback feels tough.

▪ *Health warning!* Too much conscious feedback can bring about short-term change in thinking, but a fully engaged relationship helps the client access their emotion schemes. Until the emotion schemes are felt, experienced and accessed other changes are precarious and short-lived.

▪ When addressing process, remain in touch with feeling. Move between them. Move freely between the spontaneous and reflexive. Extend your empathy to be in touch with both aspects of your client.

---

## Emotion Schemes

Emotions are best viewed as involving *action tendencies* that arise as a function of *automatic appraisals* of the relevance of situations to our *basic concerns*.

(Greenberg *et al.*, 1993, p. 49)

We do not store emotions inside us, in spite of such powerful images as our being constipated with constricted rage. Rather, we store emotion schemes. These are patterns made up of primary affects and often laid down in early life. Rogers' notion of a condition of worth refers to a species of emotion schemes. When we have an emotion, therefore, we do not consult a library of possible emotions, but use a small number of familiar schemes to guide us in constructing an emotional response to a situation.

This is a highly efficient way of being, in evolutionary terms. Emotions help us to survive by showing us how to respond to situations. We need to feel quickly and out-of-focused-awareness. Emotions are spontaneous rather than reflexive for the most part – although there will be exceptions, not least in therapy.

Gendlin's (1981) 'felt-sense' is pre-conscious emotion that manifests itself in the body, but not yet in the reflexive self-consciousness.

To return to Greenberg's quotation above, he claims that when we experience an emotion it guides us towards doing, is an action tendency and is based on an automatic, out-of-awareness assessment of the situation in terms of our basic life concerns and patterns.

Emotions tend to be highly functional experiences. However, sometimes the way we put them together is distorted, in just the way that conditions of worth distort our own self-evaluating process.

Greenberg posits three levels of processing emotions (Greenberg *et al.*, 1993, pp. 51–4):

1. sensori-motor – I 're-member' body sensations. There are no propositions or ideas and recalling is often out of my control.
2. schematic memory – concrete representations (pictures) of past experience.
3. conscious thinking within my control, and building upon beliefs, rules and so forth.

We can note from this three-level model that feeling affects thinking just because it is so often logically and biologically prior to thinking. However, this does not mean that the cognitive therapists are wholly wrong, far from it. Sometimes the process works the other way round, and can in the short term be effective. Thinking – feeling processes are essentially bi-directional (Sperry, 1995).

A healthy level of symbolization of emotions (Rogers, 1957c) swings between the second and the third levels of processing, between spontaneous and reflexive experiencing.

Figure 13.1, which aims to encapsulate the whole of the paradigm, can now be read like this. In early childhood, but also in later life, our basic affective experience lays down for us a root-system of emotion schemes. These form the pattern for our emotion-experiencing. Each time there is an event to which we need to respond emotionally, these schemes determine (to some degree) how we construe – put together in ourselves – the emotions which we then think of as coming from the trigger event. The idea of 'needing to have an emotional response' is about evolutionary need. Emotion is a swift and mainly out-of-awareness assessing of a critical situation, which demands spontaneous – that is, fast – response. Emotion only comes fully into awareness through reflexive processes which in turn slow down the reaction.

The thinking process has interrelated but logically independent schemata. These are not easy to access. To the extent that they need to change, they are better accessed through emotional experiencing.

By way of summary, we can say that cognitive schemata govern our ways of understanding. Experiencing in the here and now helps us become more flexible, but cognitive schemata are still resistant to change.

Emotion schemes are generally out of awareness. They determine how we put together our emotions in the present moment. We tend to feel now as we have felt in the past. Emotion schemes are changed by accessing feelings in the here and now and then moving forward in our felt-meaning (Gendlin, 1997). This has a large impact upon our thinking. People change most readily when their feelings are accessed to change emotion schemes. This is done through offering new experience. Only then will thinking move.

Emotion is a swift, efficient and out-of-awareness, problem-solving mechanism. It is based on parallel processing. *It is only fast and efficient because it is out of awareness.*

---

**Personal Focus 13.5    Using the diagram**

- Recall a piece of client work which is complete or nearing an ending. Be aware of the client's journey in your work together. Be aware also of your own journey and of your understanding which has come through supervision.
- Begin to map your client's change onto the diagram.
- Remember that each emotionally significant event is a new experience – the process repeats time and again, sometimes swiftly.
- When was your client most in touch with her emotion schemes/ basic affect patterns/conditions of worth and so forth?
- How did thinking change?
- How has the client changed her 'internal' story or meaning as therapy has gone on? (See Chapter 5.)

---

## A Four-stage Model of Humanistic Therapy

The point of therapy is not to use reason or evidence to change purely cognitive schemes (Beck, 1976; Ellis, 1962). Rather, it is to change the complex cognitive, affective, motivational, and relational action components of emotion schemes. Thus, an emotion scheme that generates, for example, disappointment in relation to lack of support, involves not only the expectational belief that 'no one will be there for me'. It also involves an action tendency such as to withdraw and curl up into a self-protective ball, a feeling such as emptiness in the pit of the stomach, and a desire to be comforted.

(Greenberg *et al.*, 1993, p. 67)

Greenberg *et al.* (1993) put forward a generalized model of humanistic therapy. I put it forward with the sole comment that it does seem to represent much of my own experience of person-centred work and parallels in part Rogers (1957c):

(i) attend to the experience of responding to the immediate situation. Attend to your own feelings.
(ii) symbolize it accurately – 'I feel afraid'; 'I feel like I used to when I was a child'; 'I feel as if I am trapped in a coal-mine.'
(iii) construct a complex, situational meaning. 'When I feel afraid, I feel useless. When my sister feels afraid, she says she just has to do something.'
(iv) generate an adaptive response – for instance, work out where my pattern comes from, or recognize that I can feel fear when I am with trustworthy people. Perhaps I am trustworthy and can keep myself safe.

Stage four of the model is aimed at his highly technical eclectic approach. The job of the therapist is to construct selectively for, and with, the client an appropriate treatment leading to an appropriate response. This is clearly not person-centred. Yet, for those of us who will risk following, however nervously, the Rogerian hypothesis that the six conditions of therapy are sufficient as well as necessary for the inauguration of significant, psychological change, this model seems to describe what I recognize as the client's journey, both on a small scale of a few minutes and on a large scale of a number of months.

I note that in symbolizing feeling and in constructing meaning, attention to process is just as important as attention to feeling, at least for some clients. We need to let the client's wisdom guide us as to whether we focus on feeling or process.

## Awareness and Symbolization

We only have full access to our emotion when we symbolize it (Rogers, 1967, p. 154). The paradigm sets up for us the double idea that thinking and feeling must be in dialogue, and that this dialogue can only happen in a social setting.

I want to quote Greenberg *et al.* (1993) at some length:

This integration [of the client's inner, phenomenological reality with her ability to construct meaning] will include a view of human beings as multiple level processors of different types of propositional (symbolic/ logical) and non-propositional (sensory/perceptual) information, who construct their conscious views of self and reality in a moment-by-moment fashion depending upon what they attend to.

In this view, experience depends upon the controlled, conscious, serial, conceptual processing of information, and upon the automatic, parallel processing of self-relevant information which occurs out of awareness.

An adequate theory must recognise two sources of experience, a conscious, deliberate, reflexive conceptual process (thinking) and an automatic, direct, schematic emotional process (feeling), and the constructive, dialectical relationship between them.

In this framework, a view of the bringing of previously denied material into awareness is replaced by a view of the dialectical construction of meaning.
(Greenberg *et al.*, 1993, p. 55)

Greenberg *et al.* here argue that the way we process – serial and conscious versus parallel and unconscious; symbolic and logical versus sensory and perceptual – is a biological given which requires that change involves a dialogue between these processes.

This book suggests strongly that the client will know whether she needs to address one process or another, or the process of dialogue itself. The job of the therapist is to be sensitive to this, to listen, for it is part of the client's frame of reference. At times the therapist may dare to challenge the client's preferred way of processing. Challenge is challenge to explore, not to correct. In spite of Rennie (1998), the client does have expertise in her own process.

## The Key Contribution of the Paradigm

I end with the final words of the theoretical part of Greenberg *et al.* (1993). It is the task of person-centred practitioners to work out for themselves in practice how much the paradigm informs their understanding; how much it informs their practice; how much it is alien to their way of being.

In summary, the combination of safety and process facilitation leads to a change in manner of processing for the therapy client. This includes broadening attentional allocation and perceptual structuring, facilitating memory reorganization and meaning construction, and providing new emotional and relational experience. Schematic change occurs by bringing the schematic modules into awareness. This makes them accessible to new information and reorganization, exposes them to new experience, and fosters the client's awareness of how their own schematic structures guide their views, thereby helping them to gain some control over their own construals.

(Greenberg *et al.*, 1993, p. 95)

I firmly reject for my own practice the idea that specific dysfunctions need specific interventions. To be person-centred is to work with the hypothesis that the six conditions are necessary and sufficient, in the sense outlined above in Chapters 2 and 3. The therapist's development of a treatment programme is for me clearly outside of this hypothesis.

I similarly reject Rennie's more modest claim that the therapist is an expert on the client's process, while the client is an expert on her own content and feelings. This is an unnecessary splitting. As a therapist, I note that I do have some expertise in relating and in knowing and recognizing and talking usefully about feeling. Some clients seem at first quite inept in this. However, the client is always an expert on her own feelings.

Similarly, as a therapist I do know something about client-process, but I know it experientially, I know it as a prelude to true dialogue and not as a block of knowledge to be bequeathed to the unenlightened client. Clients really are the experts in their own process. They know – as at first I certainly do not – how they react, process, deal with situations. I follow, reflect and track their processing. At times I find that I judge their process as somehow askew. I need to learn to trust it rather than to want to change it. The client will then be freed to change it if need be.

## Into Practice

The case of Hilary, below, provided me with a problem in how I thought about the therapy we were engaged in. Hilary carried a number of very painful and undermining scripts (emotion schemes and cognitive schemata, mainly top-down, concept-driven schemata). Gradually, the course of therapy eased her distress, and she came to see the part that her mother had played in distorting the life of her sisters and herself. However, in the presence of her boss, who much reminded her of her mother, she would lose any sense of self-control and composure, and be overtaken with panic and tears that disabled her as a professional. What could I do to help? We found that instructing her to call to mind a mantra about the impact upon her of her mother was useful. We practised it in therapy. Was I true to my model or had a moved into a small piece of CBT?

The paradigm is rich but complicated. The case of Hilary helped me to think through what exactly I was doing. It serves also as a fairly simple illustration of one aspect of the paradigm.

### Case 13.1  Hilary – a paradigmatic moment

*This material is used with Hilary's permission, but, more than that, this chapter has been read by her, corrected in a number of details, and then, to my fascination, shared with one of her sisters. It has turned out to be a piece of family therapy in miniature.*

Hilary has been in therapy with me for nearly two years. While we are not, as I write, very close to an ending, she has made much progress.

The details of her work within herself are not very important to this paradigm-moment. It is sufficient to say that her experience of being her mother's child has been negative and painful. Mother left her with the deeply ingrained sense of being unsatisfactory. (Mother did this to all of her children, and has left them in a state of frozen sibling rivalry which is only just beginning to emerge within the family in the middle years of life.) Hilary has believed herself to be unsatisfactory in many ways. The harsh conditions of worth with which she has lived have left her with a strong belief in her life as self-defeating. In moments of closeness it is bound, she thinks, to go wrong. That is how she is.

While there is a distinct fragility to Hilary when she is in touch with this life-script, she is far from being a rigid person. I find her warm, emotionally very much alive, talented, although sometimes dismissive of her own abilities. She has an immediacy in relating that I experience as profoundly authentic. She has a lively sense of humour and can laugh at herself as well as others. Laughter is part of the therapeutic process. I use my own sense of mischief to 'address ironically' (gently, I hope) her scripty self-misperceptions, now that we are well into our work. It is risky at times, yet it gives congruent perspective to her and her mother-bequeathed aspects. Above all, Hilary is a skilled and gifted worker with people. She has the ability to persevere in areas of life, and with her own and others' pain, when many would become despondent.

Her belief that she is of low worth and 'a problem' has led her in the past to introject others' criticisms, verbal or attitudinal. This is now receding. It had made relating problematical for her, whenever the relationship involved intimacy.

I note with particular interest that Hilary has throughout our work together tended to need and want to conceptualize her patterns, her introjects, her conditions of worth, the links between past and present. I note from a number of years as a person-centred therapist that some clients clearly seek to conceptualize, while others seem either to have no need to or are perhaps even unable to conceptualize their own process. This is a key issue for me. Rogers' (1957a) description of the therapeutic process is perfectly clear that a making-conscious of the process is not necessary for therapeutic change. I do not dissent from this. Clients seem to me to choose. I have come to believe that the need to conceptualize is sometimes very much an expression of the organism's healthy and preferred way of working. I need, as therapist, to be open to whichever is the appropriate process for any given client.

## The Client's Preferred Way of Working – an Excursus

When I work with a natural conceptualizer like Hilary, I can sometimes feel ill at ease. By contrast, when all change is out of focused awareness then I am sure that I am working true to the person-centred approach. At the risk of parodying the latter case, I can see good psychotherapy in action, while the client feels better because of 'our little chats'. (There is, of course, a cultural element in how clients conceive of their therapy.) But with conceptualizers, I need continually to monitor what I am doing.

If the client is operating at the cognitive level for some parts of the therapy, I need to check out with myself that I am not wandering into a sort of cognitive therapy. If the client values insight, I can facilitate her in acquiring it, but I may not give it, as from above. The boundary here is fine and difficult. Interpreting is the strong suggesting of meaning or connections. To interpret is not so much a use of words as a use of power. Phenomenological exploration is the self-consciously puzzled opening-up of the way the client's process, meaning, feelings and life events interact.

Hilary, as conceptualizer, has a keen notion of her internal dialogues. Cognitive therapy sees this dialogue as easily accessible, and therefore the key way to change irrational thinking and hence the emotions that follow it. Hilary certainly might want to describe her misrepresentations of herself to herself as 'irrational thinking'. However, the paradigm points to the key fact that cognitive schemata are difficult to modify, with concept-driven schemata being less flexible than data-driven schemata. They are the result of, rather than the cause of, emotional experience, which itself is created anew with each piece of experiencing on the basis of the emotion schemes which are laid down in early life.

In order to avoid 'becoming cognitive', I need to pay full empathic attention to Hilary's thinking and her self-conceptualizing of the 'messages' from mother, and at the same time also remain fully aware of the relationship between Hilary's thinking, her emotions and the underlying affect schemes (in Rogers' terms, her conditions of worth). In order to avoid the cognitive therapy pitfall, the tempting short cut, I need first to maintain empathy with all parts of Hilary's process, much as we have seen Mearns maintaining empathy with each configuration of Elizabeth. Secondly, I will remain alert to cognition as being largely derivative of emotion schemes. Thirdly, I will attempt to explore the client's phenomenology of her own structuring of experience if that seems an appropriate form of empathy.

This phenomenological commitment is then the key to avoiding interpretation. It is possible that the client and I can explore how she puts together her experience. I can even test out empathically some of my perceptions which derive in part from theorizing as well as observing – what Mearns and Thorne call 'depth reflection' (Mearns and Thorne, 2007, pp. 71 & 78). Yet, phenomenological exploring is always open to the client's primary experiencing and her willingness or otherwise to own my empathic reflections on her experience. My work with Hilary will illustrate these points.

## Working with Hilary – the Paradigm-Moment

My experience of Hilary in the early days of therapy had been that her emotions, her tears, were overwhelming. They seemed to me like a plunge into an abyss of despair. In more recent sessions, she has still been able to contact this level of experiencing, but it has been more under her control. She can both fully experience her emotions and at the same time reflect upon them. This is a major step forward for her in what Rogers (1957c) terms the symbolizing of experience. I note that, with growing awareness, it is likely that Hilary will move this process of symbolization from the reflexive towards the spontaneous pole of her experiencing. In other words, her reflection will become faster, less conscious and more connected to a helpful felt-sense of her own well-being. The final instants of this paradigm-moment show signs of this beginning to happen.

The movement of process of difficult feeling from the reflexive to the spontaneous is a phenomenon I frequently encounter. This is part of the evolutionary aspect of the brain and the psyche. The faster we can process, the more functional we are. However, there is a fine line to walk here. Good functioning is available to consciousness; fast functioning is generally out of awareness, just to the degree that it is based on parallel rather than serial processing. (See above.)

I suggest that healthy functioning is therefore congruent with this tension. It is in part spontaneous and in part reflexive. There is a struggle for balance. This struggle can be seen as explaining why no person is perfectly functional. To be fully functioning is, both in Rogers' (1957b) sense and in process terms, to be processing this tension creatively. By way of example, I experience myself as functioning well when I can both live in the present moment and also be reflectively aware of what matters to me in my experience.

Meaning, and our ability to express this as narrative, requires us to be both spontaneous and reflexive. When we are spontaneous, we are in touch with our felt-sense of what things mean (Gendlin, 1997) and when we are reflexive we are self-conscious tellers of our own story.

Hilary arrived for our session looking concerned. She had a relatively new relationship with Gregory. It felt like light at the end of a lonely tunnel. Gregory's mother had been showing signs of frailty over the past months. Now, it was apparent that she would come to live with Gregory. Their relationship was not far enough on for this to warrant consultation, for that would have presumed too much. For Hilary, this felt devastating.

She told me of the new arrangements, reminding me, quite calmly, of some details that had slipped my mind. Then, almost as if by way of summary, she commented that it was all going wrong again. I remained with her feeling of growing despair. She began to weep copiously. I allowed myself just a couple of minutes to remain with her overwhelming feelings. I needed to convey that I knew the pain was strong and real. Since I was about to challenge its basis, I gave particular attention to acknowledging the force and intensity of this experience.

Hilary commented that it felt just the same as always. It was bound to go wrong. I observed, as if in parallel to her own comment, that this must feel familiar territory to her. Gradually, she reached the point of being able to recite her mother's messages. She would never have a satisfactory relationship with a man. (That was her role in the birth-family; to carry her mother's feelings of relational ineptitude.)

I felt as if I was walking a tightrope between feeling and process. I wanted to remain in touch with the waves of despair and grief. If I were to let go of these, so might Hilary. I knew that they were, as you might say, supposed to be there. To lose focus on the emotion is to risk invoking a defence against fully experiencing feeling. On the other hand, there are also moments when the client seems to be drowning in her emotion. Process work can be a compensatory move towards the reflexive pole. The basic skill of process work is to be in touch with both emotion and process. Symbolization of experience requires both. In the end, this is what the client is to do for herself.

What I most readily noticed about Hilary at this point was her new-found ability to relate her story with calm, and then to begin to contact her feelings, however devastating they felt as they formed within her. As yet, her feelings still threaten to swamp her listening to them at the very moment they happen. This listening process – empathy with the self – is again a new-found competence for Hilary. It will, I believe, become more readily available. Feelings will be both more fully experienced and more fully symbolized (Rogers, 1957c). This represents the balance and tension between the spontaneous and the reflexive.

We moved between the feelings and Hilary's awareness of the maternal messages. This movement from one to the other deserves much comment. It seems to me to be at the heart of person-centred process work. The risk of process work is that it takes the client away from their feelings. Good process work can also stay with feelings. It is important to remain with clients' feelings for as much of process work as possible.

Process work is a form of empathy. Rogers (1951) sees empathy very much as search for understanding and clarification of the client's internal frame of reference (Rogers, 1951, pp. 26–30). This does not always mean working in depth with feelings. I can empathize in depth with my client's process as well as with her emotions; 'is this how you are coming to experience yourself?'

However, the movement between feelings and process seems to me to resemble the fourth of Gendlin's focusing movements – resonating the handle (Gendlin, 1981, pp. 56–7). In this, Gendlin has already invited the client to experience the felt-sense and then to begin to symbolize it by struggling (internal empathy) to name it accurately. The symbolizing process is deepened by moving swiftly between the felt-sense and the handle (the name). Hilary's ability to move swiftly between distressing emotion and her insight into it is analogous. She is beginning to symbolize her internal world more accurately and critically. This in turn allows her to internalize her locus of evaluation (Mearns and Thorne, 1999, pp. 10–12).

After a while, a link seemed to have been experienced. The depth of emotion began to subside. At the point that I might have felt that a particular movement of therapy had come to an end, I was intensely grateful for a flash of insight. I stood back a little way and took a broader perspective: 'It must be really difficult for someone like you that as you change you have to learn for a while to distrust your own feelings.'

This seemed an odd comment for a therapist. Surely we ought to trust what we feel? Hilary is a creative, artistic and deeply intuitive person. She listens deeply and I guess has a reserve of natural empathy. In her daily work with others she trusts her feelings in learning what is happening for those for whom she cares. She is professionally orientated to know and trust what she feels. Yet at trigger moments in her life her emotions are untrustworthy. They are out of date. They are the presenting past.

Her contacting the familiarity of recognizing this and resonating it with the raw feeling itself seems to me to be a core part of her healing. She was doing just that, moreover, more and more independently of me. I attempted to extend empathy to this process. It must be hard to find the tunedness of one's own emotions becoming so cacophonous!

To my delight, she contradicted me. No! Not all of her emotions felt untrustworthy. Not even at those trigger moments. Sometimes she had a very great sense of the truth of what she felt. She did after all know when her emotions were congruent with a healthier version of her self-concept and when they were contaminated by the maternal voice.

I searched for the right image: 'it is as if a part of you really has been a trustworthy companion even in the darkest moments of the journey'. This she could own.

The empathic nature of process work was marked out by my need to find an image that would embody my response to her process, and in particular her healthy processing. The fact of a trustworthy, lifelong companion within the self is Hilary's radical discovery – and is yet to be developed more fully – but the picture of it is my response to listening in depth to her. It is, as Rogers (1986b) notes, governed by the underlying question of all empathic responding:

> Is this the way it is in you? Am I catching just the color and texture and flavor of the personal meaning you are experiencing right now?
>
> (Rogers, 1986b, cited in Kirschenbaum and Henderson, 1990a, p. 128)

## Process Work in Action

Hilary's conditions of worth were set in her at two different levels. Her mother had imbued in her a number of interlocking cognitive schemata concerning her alleged inadequacy as a person in relationship, as a woman and as someone engaged in a hopeless quest for a partner. The schemata were firmly embedded; that is to say, they were concept-driven and so reluctant to change. Connected with these, but separate in terms of triggers, were a number of emotion schemes which, in adverse circumstances, would generate in Hilary an overwhelming sense of distress and self-disgust. This disabled her in relating and even in conversing. These schemes could be triggered by harsh challenge, by conflict, by rejection, but also by desire and by the admiration and approval of others.

I am sometimes struck by the fact that the cognitive schemata and emotion schemes which make up our conditions of worth often are structured self-protectively, and mirror the double-binds by which we have been ensnared in the first place. Thus, Hilary could experience the internal shift of emotions in therapy, in response to my acceptance and empathy, but this was then disabled by the mother-driven cognitive schemata cutting in across it. What could disrupt this?

I have described Hilary as needing to conceptualize her own process. This she seemed to know, at least in part. It felt useful to her. In so doing, she began to give herself cognitive feedback to lay down a number of rather fragile – at first – data-driven, or bottom-up, schemata. These she could recycle to cut across the rigidity of the conceptual schemata that represent the internalized aspects of her critical mother. In other words, the new, data-driven schemata were able to move Hilary from out-of-awareness, serial processing with its cascade of negative affect and thinking, towards a more reflexive stance in which she was able to intervene with herself. Only as her self-trust grew could she return to a more spontaneous way of living, balanced against the necessary reflexivity.

As the whole structure began to find a new looseness, a responsiveness to good experience and consequent increase in self-trusting, Hilary was able to intuit that she had all along been a good-enough companion to herself. In other words, even when she was at her most self-denigrating, there was an unconscious engagement with her organismic value process in the form (or under the metaphor) of self-accompaniment.

Both in the flow of therapy and in retrospect, theoretical models inform what we do and how it engages the client constructively.

## Further Reading

Baker, N. (2004) 'Experiential Person-Centred Therapy'. In P. Sanders (ed.) *The Tribes of the Person-Centred Nation: An Introduction to the Schools of Therapy Related to the Person-Centred Approach*. Ross-on-Wye, PCCS Books, pp. 67–94.
Baker, N. (2007) *The Experiential Counselling Primer*. Ross-on-Wye, PCCS Books.

Nick Baker is the pre-eminent British practitioner of the person-centred, process-experiential model. His approach is useful, responsible, scholarly and very approachable. His work is the easiest way into further consideration of process-experiential work.

Greenberg, L.S., L.N. Rice and R. Elliott (1993) *Facilitating Emotional Change: The Moment-by-Moment Process*. New York, The Guilford Press.

This is a book of the utmost importance in that its roots in research as well as practice are impeccable. However, it is a book of two halves. The theory in the first 95 pages is invaluable. However, what is deduced from it – and called a 'treatment manual' within the book – is based upon the specificity myth.

Lietaer, G. (1998) 'From Non-Directive to Experiential: A Paradigm Unfolding' in Thorne and Lambers, 62–73.

A brief and scholarly introduction to the process-experiential paradigm from a European perspective.

# 14

# Process Work in Practice

> The human person deeply desires expression. One of the most beautiful ways the soul is present is through thought. Thoughts are the forms of the soul's inner swiftness .... Our feelings too can move swiftly; yet even though they are precious to our own identity, thoughts and feelings still remain largely invisible. In order to feel real, we need to bring that inner, invisible world to expression.
>
> (O'Donohue, 1997, p. 170)

The words of John O'Donohue make for me deep intuitive connections with all manner of lived experience. In the passage above from his *Anam Cara* he is speaking of work. Some work certainly does not 'bring the inner, invisible world to expression'. The mindlessness of industrial alienation in which the profit motive drives those with power to demand more and more of those who offer their labour is literally soul-destroying; industry is wise to attempt to move away from this version of mass production to a more humane and humanistic view of work.

I feel fortunate to be both a priest and a therapist, for in each role my own work echoes the words of O'Donohue. I am present as others bring their being to expression.

For person-centred therapists, it is at the core of our convictions that the person of our client strives and yearns to express its inwardness in the swift movement of feeling and thinking and thence into the storied actions in the world by which we constitute ourselves. We often speak of what the client does as 'work'. It much resembles work in O'Donohue's far more general sense of the word. I note with delight that the qualities that mark the client's work, the client's process towards increasing functionality, also represent what I call my job satisfaction and my spirituality of counselling.

It is when the client can express her precious identity that I too express mine. These are not parallel processes, the one contaminating the other. I do not feed parasitically on my client, but rather her nourishing of herself is also

228

the partial expression of my identity. My being in the presence of her act of growth is self-expression by me.

At this most general of levels, I come to recognize that the client and I share an aspiration spoken from our actualizing tendency to become who we are and in this we share in a humanity which transcends divisions between selves and within the self. We meet no longer as individuals but as those who participate in community.

These underlying values which I hope suffuse the detail of this book express themselves in particular when I am open to my client's process.

The final chapter of a book might attempt to summarize what has gone before and to look to future developments. Yet this is the pattern of *knowledge*. I will make some movement in this direction, but only in the light of a deep inward protest that the heart of process working is not knowledge, but *wisdom*. Wisdom is in the integration of a sort of experiential knowing into the fullness of our own humanity.

Process work has always been for me a combination of three qualities:

1. On the surface, I can describe my client's process and make decisions about how I will contact it. I can take this to supervision. I can analyse my own thinking and processing about this. Yet in this there is the danger that I relate to her process as an I–It. My thinking objectifies what I see and removes me from it. If our practice remains at this level, then it is so much dross.

2. At the level of the imagination, as I sit before and with my client, I can picture, model and strive for some symbolization of her processing, with the conviction that this is an act of deep empathy. If my client were physically transparent, then I would see, and she would see, her internal organs alive and functioning. This could be a strange and even invasive experience. It would need to be grasped as a shared and respectful gazing, and an openness to its beauty. I sometimes picture empathy-with-process as a striving for mental transparency, in which together she and I gaze at her self-expressing humanity in its tentativeness and detail; in its woundedness and hesitancy; in its vitality and fluency.

3. At the third level, when I meet my client's process, her self, I encounter my own humanity. This is phenomenologically rooted spirituality. It is as if speech about this feels increasingly futile, but if I lose a sense of therapy as sacred space then I run the risk of abusing the fragile openness of my client; it would be the abuse of failing to perceive the radical Otherness of those whom I meet in community.

In this concluding chapter, I will suggest by way of summary something of the nature of process-engagement at each of these three levels.

# Level One – The Arguments

**Personal Focus 14.1   Check your understanding**

*The first level of process work is expressed as a series of proposi-
tions. Use these to check your understanding of this book.*

- Process work in person-centred therapy can be located across
  a range of primary and secondary principles, in accord with
  Sanders' Chicago 2000 position statement. It can range along a
  continuum that stretches from the literalist to the experientialist
  extremes.
- Process work does not necessarily involve a shift in the therapist's
  role, *pace* Rennie (1998).
- Process work is best conceived of as depth reflection, and hence
  an expression or instantiation of the core conditions of therapy.
- Process work is not necessarily any more directive than classical person-centred work. It can aspire to abide by the secondary
  as well as the primary principles of the Chicago 2000 position
  statement.
- All work is directive to the extent that the therapist has no choice
  but to choose between reflecting the known content of the client's
  self-expression and working with her process as self-expression.
- Process is one aspect of the client's frame of reference. To ignore
  it in practice is to be unempathic. To decline to engage with it
  on principle is to reject the holistic nature of the person-centred
  tradition.
- Person-Centred therapy needs to be grounded in a practical
  and theoretical grasp of phenomenology. This includes the key
  observation that we need to function both spontaneously and
  reflexively.
- The client's process can be symbolized in therapy by either the
  client or the therapist. This symbolization can be enriched by
  access to the resources of much of humanistic thinking: narrative, metaphor, ego-states, awareness and its interruption are but
  examples.
- Consequently, it is possible to integrate theory without compro-
  mising the principles of person-centred therapy (Sanders, 2000,
  p. 70). Integration of theory does not imply integration of practice
  and certainly not eclecticism.
- A depth of grasp of the phenomenological principle frees the
  therapist into a practice that is truly personal, even idiosyncratic,

and certainly not bound up with a rigid conception of person-centredness.

The same principle is also a key to perceiving the project of therapy as spiritual in a way that is open to religious and non-religious spiritualities alike.

Person-Centred practice is in essence phenomenological. It is arguably also existential..

Existentialist thinking suggests that the primacy of relating is ontological as well as empirical in its basis (Buber, 1958). It is about encountering the Other, the human and perhaps, with Buber and Levinas, the divine, both of which are radically beyond the self.

Existentialist thinking raises a large number of questions that might be subsumed under the general question of authenticity. The therapist is called by this to face the judgement that might be raised against those clients who live, by apparent choice, inauthentically.

When clients can 'hold' their own processing as both spontaneous and reflexive, the therapist may enter into a position that engages with the existential issues of life. Existential therapy within the person-centred tradition is sensitive to the client's ability to process autonomously.

Because process work is empathy at depth, it benefits from an act of imagination in both the client and the therapist. The work in practice can be fine-tuned by reference to useful paradigms of process (Greenberg *et al.*, 1993).

Treat all that goes before as useful hypothesis and then learn from the client (Rogers, 1951; Casement, 1985, 1990).

## Level Two – Process: Imaging and Imagination

Gestalt theory describes three zones of experiencing: outer, inner and middle (Sills *et al.*, 1995, p. 27). The first two correspond approximately with the outer world and the embodied self. The middle zone is the point of contact between these, and is a mental phenomenon populated with images, fantasies, self-talk and the like. The contents of the middle zone can interrupt the flow of experiencing or they can facilitate it. Because the client's process is often out of the client's focused awareness, the role of the therapist, in listening to this aspect of the client's frame of reference, is often to resonate between close phenomenological attention to the client's feelings and body-language and an openness to her own imaging of the client's process.

This can be illustrated from a moment of Carl Rogers' work with Kathy (Rogers, 1977):

---

**Box 14.1   Kathy's silence**

Kathy has been describing to Rogers her ambivalent feelings about the death of her husband from whom she was separated. It was for her the loss of a safety mechanism. She feared intimacy with other men and, as long as he was alive, she felt protected from this possibility. She was afraid of commitment: 'How can you be lovers without being friends first?' After a while she stopped speaking, her face hardened a little and she drew back in her chair. There was a silence.

Rogers first noticed the process. She had been talking about relating with him. She had then come to an end. He offered empathy to this process. It was as if she wanted to go no further. Why should he be allowed to get closer to her? 'Damn it! Stay away from me.'

---

## Reflection

At this point in his relationship with Kathy, Rogers is both intuitive and deeply empathic; he is in touch with, and is imaging within himself, her process, but might be described as strongly interpretative. Rogers was not immune from interpretation! (Farber *et al.*, 1996, pp. 21, 84–94). From my perspective, Rogers experiences a switch within himself from his focused attention being on Kathy's feelings to a point where he is increasingly aware of her process. This may have been growing within him for a number of minutes, but clearly affects his behaviour only as he addresses Kathy's silence.

The act of imaging or of imagination within Rogers is to allow himself to picture the immediate experience of the therapy room as an expression of 'what Kathy does'. The process of Kathy and of Kathy-and-Carl-together has been present in the room from the very beginning. The switch occurs when Carl allows this process to enter his awareness as the predominant figure, and then acts upon this perception. Rogers offers the observation that Kathy wants to go no further with him either. It is as if she does this all the time (in particular with men). In psychodynamic terms, he points to and then gently interprets the transference.

Why do I insist that this is an act of imagination?

To return to basic principles, the person-centred practitioner aspires to avoid being directive in principle, and eschews interpreting the transference. Yet it looks as if this is what Rogers does here. The person-centred approach is based upon the therapeutic value of relating, upon the necessity and sufficiency of the core conditions and upon trust in the client's (and therapist's) actualizing tendency. All of these qualities are long-term projects within the relationship. No small-scale intervention violates these principles in and of itself. Rogers' intervention in Kathy's silence is person-centred because it is set within the deeper qualities of his relationship with Kathy.

It is clear that a psychodynamic counsellor using the transference in the way that Rogers does here would be engaged in a long-term project of assisting Kathy in gaining insight. This might be the main motif of work. Of course person-centred therapists also help clients gain insight, but the fundamental intention of the therapist differs. I suggest that the word 'analysis' is telling. Psychodynamic therapy attempts to offer insight in matching the client's experience with preconceived theory on a large scale. Michael Jacobs describes it thus:

> However much of a client's personal history emerges, the psychodynamic approach is distinct from other models of counselling, in that the counsellor remains aware of the developmental issues described in psychodynamic theory, using these ideas to try and throw light on what a client says and in the way a client reacts to the counsellor.
>
> (Jacobs, 1988, p. 11)

The client's experience is matched against theory. The stance of the counsellor is objective. The key activity is interpretation.

Even when the activity is momentarily the same, as here with Rogers, the underlying relational stance of the therapist differs. I stress the importance of imagination in process work because I believe that the imaginative act is more true to the basic phenomenological perspective. If I think consistently about what the client is doing, matching observed fact to theory and striving to make sense of the former in terms of the latter, I have departed from the intention of the person-centred practitioner. If, on the other hand, I listen, above all listen, and then allow my intuition, my imagination, to cast up for me figures and patterns of the client's process, and if I desire no more than to understand and cherish this process, then I may stand within the intentional structure of the person-centred approach.

The act of imaging, of envisioning, the client's process is creative and not analytical. I clearly strive to understand by allowing as much of myself as I can make available to contact the client's being. I see the client-in-process as a subjective act. It is mine. I own it. I check it out with the client continually because I remain radically unsure of it. Indeed the psychodynamic practitioner will also check out that the client can own an interpretation. Yet the therapeutic process differs.

When I engage the client's process from the depths of my imaging and imagining, I work at the subjective and spontaneous end of the spectrum and am in desperate need of doubting that my seeing and the client's reality match. When I interpret as an act of matching, I work far more reflexively and may become too certain of the correspondence of my seeing to reality.

To be committed to the image-centredness of process work is to remain true to the phenomenological underpinning of our model.

## Images and Paradigms

The experience of watching repeatedly, and with many groups of students, the few moments in which Rogers addresses Kathy's silence and his mode of dealing with this as transference is linked for me with my own experience of being with clients at key moments of their processing. Person-Centred therapists need to image/imagine the client's process, so that this imaging is thoroughly and intuitively embedded in the therapist's own felt-awareness. It is then available to be treated tentatively and offered back to the client as depth reflection, a striving after empathic contact rather than as authoritative interpretation. It is crucial to the instantiation of the core conditions that the client's process is imaged. It is metaphor, alive with excess meaning but also untrustworthy at the cognitive level, and so to be offered back diffidently.

What is true of individual moments of actual process is the case *a fortiori* with models and paradigms of process. The paradigm outlined very briefly in Chapter 13 is also an image, but this time an image that might apply to all processing. It is generalized, but not thereby any more 'authoritative'. The therapist must still use her imaging with respect, diffidence, caution and care. Nothing is *known* from the paradigm, but only suggested, as a possible way of conceptualizing experience.

## Into Practice

To illustrate what has just been said, I return to the case of Hilary described in Chapter 13.

I was becoming aware that Hilary carries a pattern of emotion schemes which is particularly toxic. The primitive schemes involve her in feeling, but only as a felt-sense, that she is profoundly untrustworthy. This is triggered in particular when she faces a double-bind set by her mother. These include attempts to succeed in sexual relationships and her commitment to her work. These triggers result in the formation afresh, time and again, of emotions of despair and catastrophe and, as I am only just beginning to grasp fully, many months later, feelings of self-disgust. In turn, her thought patterns are self-defeating ones. She knows with certainty that she may not succeed, because when she tries to the result is self-disgust. (The actual pattern is more complex than this, but this will suffice.) Therefore, Hilary had developed a life story in which the dominating theme was that she could not trust her feelings with men because this would lead to self-rejection. It had become fixed as a cognitive schema, which then became a self-fulfilling prophecy.

Cognitive therapists might like to reflect upon the fact that the paradigm, put forward by Greenberg *et al.*, 1993, does offer an accurate image of my experience of Hilary; to assail the thinking is pointless, for the defences are far too subtle and circular. The roots are deeper. They subsist in the way the emotions put themselves together on each occasion.

The *blik*, the moment of revelation in which Hilary and I recognized that the ensnarement was not complete, occurred when she was able to feel as felt-sense that not all of her emotions following trigger-situations were any longer unreliable. Enough of her subterranean structure had shifted unseen in therapy for us both to be astonished that she had become more functional. We have developed an image for this: she now has a place to stand which is safe, and in which she can *observe* her processing.

Hilary and I have come to know, to be familiar with and befriend, her processing, both cognitively and intuitively. The beginning of the process was spontaneous and out of the awareness of both of us. It has now become reflexive for both of us. The switch-moment was my empathic challenge: it must be difficult for Hilary not to trust her emotional responses (in trigger situations), when they are so reliable at other times. In its reflexivity, it became available to Hilary in a new way. She could process cognitively her new patterns and abilities. Her new cognitive schemata were rooted in the experience of therapy to such a degree that they were flexible, bottom–up, open to experience and hence more functional.

However, having described some of the links between Hilary-in-process and the Greenberg paradigm, I want to raise a question. Did I have Greenberg in mind? I am sure that the answer is that at no point in my work did Greenberg's paradigm cross my mind. Sometimes in therapy a theoretical perspective will rear its head. On this occasion it did not. It is possible, of course, that the paradigm is wholly *post factum*, that it did no more than help me understand where we had been, a piece of internal supervision. This is not, I believe, the case.

I suggest that part of reflective practice involves the integration of theoretical insight into the spontaneous, out-of-focused-awareness, intuitive and image-generating part of the therapist. I cannot demonstrate it even subjectively, but I deeply suspect that theoretical insights, when integrated by the mature practitioner, not only inform the reflexive mind, but equip the spontaneous being of the therapist.

## Level Three – Process and Spiritual Awareness

I choose to describe some experiencing with clients as having a spiritual quality to it. I do not imply that this involves experiencing 'a different realm'. (I do not personally preclude that either.) Rather, I point to the spiritual as a quality of being with the client. I note that this is more readily available to us as a dyad, when at least I am in touch with the client's processing as well as other aspects of her frame of reference. I suspect that this is so because process work, if it is not to be 'analytical', is a deeper act of imagination and imaging. In it I sense something of the holistic nature of my client. I could of course leave the matter there and let the reader say merely that Richard labours under the illusion that, when he is in touch with the client's process, he is in touch with a deeper element of the client – which is certainly the case – and that this element is qualitatively spiritual – which is not at all obvious. How might we move beyond this veneer that the quality of spiritual significance is just in the eye of the beholder?

I am much indebted here to the argument of a superb article, 'Unconditional Positive Regard and Its Spiritual Implications' by Campbell Purton (1998). Purton offers an ingenious way forward, which at least provides a parallel and context to my own claim that process work contributes to the awareness of the spiritual in therapy.

Purton heads his article with a quotation from the Catholic existentialist, Gabriel Marcel:

> *Aimer un être, c'est lui dire: Toi, tu ne mourras pas.*
> To love someone is to say to her: You will not know death.
> (Thorne and Lambers, 1998, p. 23)

The basic force of his argument is that unconditional respect can seem to be a sentimental attitude, particularly since there are real problems in separating the deed from the person in the way often suggested. In other words, there seem to be no convincing empirical grounds for according unconditional respect to persons. Therefore if the notion of unconditional respect is to have any force, it will be as a transcendental notion: people deserve it purely by virtue of being people. Hence, the words of Marcel suggest that, in loving someone and therefore desiring their immortality in more than a sentimental way, we are in touch with that person as essential rather than empirical self. There are many religious versions of this transcendental argument: for instance, we are worthy of respect without condition because we are made in the image of God. However, Purton needs a universal version of this. He opts for a version put forward by the philosopher Harry Frankfurt, a version which is particularly attractive to therapists. Frankfurt points out that people are different from animals because they have second-order desires. This is equivalent to saying that they are reflexive as well as spontaneous. A second-order desire expresses itself thus: I am always cruel but I truly desire to be different. Second-order desire resembles the notion of the actualizing tendency. Frankfurt's argument is that we are different not because we can change but because we can desire to change our desires. This means that we cannot exhaust our potential for change. This in turn is another version of Mearns' argument that the word 'evil' should never be applied to people, because they never have definitively exhausted their capacity for change (Mearns and Thorne, 2000, pp. 67–8).

Purton then notes that there are two radically different versions of his argument. The humanist version, to use his turn of phrase, is purely empirical. It happens to be a fact, because we are reflexive, that people can never in principle exhaust their potential to change, for as beings it is inherent in our natures that we have second-order desires. However, there is another version of this which states that people, if they are to receive unconditional respect, must have the capacity to transcend their empirical capacity for change in this world. There is implicit in the notion of unconditional respect a hint, a rumour, that people transcend their limited desires not only by second-order longings for change but also by having lives which are in some sense lived beyond the level of empirical reality, in which this change can be realized. Purton makes no commitment as to the nature of this essential life.

In either version of his argument, Purton is putting forward a way in which a commitment at a practical level to according unconditional respect is a spiritual commitment in the sense of the word spiritual developed in Chapter 11. In the second, transcendental, version the word spiritual can tolerate a stricter or narrower sense, hinting at links between unconditional respect and the transcendence of the material world.

Purton's argument gives context to all process work as spiritual. Harry Frankfurt's case is that what is essentially human is our reflexivity. It is my experience that in empathizing with the client's process I will often be sharing a journey towards a more reflexive awareness of that process within the client. She and I grow in reflexivity together, and are thus freed into a greater spontaneity of being.

This is to be fully functioning (Rogers, 1957b), and to be fully functioning is a matter of no small spiritual significance.

## Future Work

This book has been directed towards a practical development of reflective practice in respect of engagement with the client's process. It will inform both the classical and the experientially orientated practitioner. It points also to future work yet to be done. I suggest that this revolves about at least four key questions:

- I have argued that process work is wholly compatible with the necessity and sufficiency of the core conditions of therapy, if it is practised in a way that is mindful of the Chicago 2000 principles, and that it need be no more directive, in principle, than classical person-centred practice. This leads to the question: how does the client experience process work compared with classical interventions? This could be researched either in terms of qualitative psychotherapy outcome or through a more localized reflection such as the use of Interpersonal Process Recall. The former is difficult, because it would require the elimination of many other variables than those which characterize process work. The latter would be no more than seeking the client's view, systematically, as to which therapist interventions are felt to be more facilitative, and why or how.

- I have argued at length that process work benefits from an integration of theory from other branches of humanistic therapy and of paradigms from humanistic psychology. I have speculated that this is concerned with the imaginative resources of the therapist working largely out of awareness at least within the therapy room. What work remains to be done in the work of further theoretical integration without compromise to the primary principles of Chicago 2000? What work remains to be done in developing dialogue between classical and experiential practitioners or those process-orientated therapists who take different stances in respect of the secondary principles of Chicago 2000?

- I have argued that careful attention to the phenomenological principle that person-centred therapy shares with other therapies leads to possible commitments to the spirituality of counselling and to the existential nature of human being. The latter of these is the more controversial. Since at the heart of person-centred therapy lies therapist attitude, there is much work to be done upon the effect of the therapist's taking up these commitments. Is Rogers correct that the therapist is at her most effective when she is open to the spiritual dimension of experience? Is an awareness that some clients choose to live authentically while others do not the end of unconditional positive regard or the beginning of a new resource for both client and therapist?

- I have argued that in paying due attention to the phenomenological approach we cannot ignore what can be learned from other humanistic approaches. However, beyond the humanistic therapies lie two other traditions which demand that we explore with them their wisdom: object relations theory and group analysis. It is perhaps the case that aspects of the Greenberg paradigm provide us with a common ground for this exploration with our psychodynamic and our cognitive-behavioural colleagues.

## Conclusion

The ending of a recent book by Dave Mearns and Brian Thorne calls us to extend to ourselves as professionals and practitioners or student therapists the core conditions, so that we can affirm all that we have to offer today. They include these words:

this single motivating force in the human organism [the actualizing tendency] is more subtle and complex in its operation than we might initially imagine. We need to listen attentively to the many configurations of the Self before we know the sense of integration which comes from accessing the actualizing tendency in its unique and socially mediated complexity.

(Mearns and Thorne, 2000, p. 219)

To listen to configurations of the Self is to do process work, at least one variety. There are many others. It is to address empathically that which client and therapist together can image as happening 'within' the client. Careful attention to the process aspect of the client's frame of reference is near the heart of person-centred therapy. It is a trusting in the client, their actualizing tendency and the necessity and sufficiency of the six conditions of therapy.

# Bibliography

Adorno, T.W. (2003) *The Jargon of Authenticity*. London, Routledge.

Alberes, R.-M. (1967) *Sartre*. Paris, Editions Universitaires.

Austin, J.L. (1961) *How To Do Things with Words*. Oxford, Oxford University Press.

Baker, N. (2004) 'Experiential Person-Centred Therapy' in P. Sanders (ed.) *The Tribes of the Person-Centred Nation: An Introduction to the Schools of Therapy Related to the Person-Centred Approach*. Ross-on-Wye, PCCS Books, pp. 67–94.

Baker, N. (2008) *The Experiential Counselling Primer*. Ross-on-Wye, PCCS Books.

Barrett-Lennard, G.T. (1998) *Carl Rogers' Helping System: Journey and Substance*. London, Sage.

Bateson, G. (1973) *Steps to an Ecology of Mind*. London, Granada.

Becker, C.S. (1992) *Living and Relating: An Introduction to Phenomenology*. London, Sage.

Berne, E. (1964) *Games People Play: The Psychology of Human Nature*. Harmondsworth, Penguin.

Bentall, R.P. (2003) *Madness Explained: Psychosis and Human Nature*. Harmondsworth, Penguin.

Biermann-Ratjen, E-M. (1998) 'Incongruence and Psychopathology' in B. Thorne and E. Lambers (eds) *Person-Centred Therapy: A European Perspective*. London, Sage, pp. 119–30.

Bozarth, J. (1998) *Person-Centred Therapy: A Revolutionary Paradigm*. Ross-on-Wye, PCCS Books.

Brazier, D. (ed.) (1993) *Beyond Carl Rogers*. London, Constable.

Brodley, B.T. (1990) 'Client-Centered and Experiential: Two Different Therapies' in G. Lietaer, J. Rombauts and R. Van Balen (eds) *Client-Centered and Experiential Psychotherapy in the Nineties*. Belgium, Leuven University Press.

Brown, D. (1987) *Continental Philosophy and Modern Theology*. Oxford, Basil Blackwell.

Buber, M. (1958) *I and Thou*. Edinburgh, T & T Clark.

Buber, M. (1961) *Between Man and Man*. London, Collins/Fontana.

Buber, M. (1991) *Tales of the Hasidim* (in two volumes). London, Random House, Schocken Books.

Bugental, J.F.T. (1954) 'The Third Force in Psychology' in *Journal of Humanistic Psychology* 4:1, pp. 19–25.

Cain, D. (ed.) (2002) *Classics in the Person-Centred Approach*. Ross-on-Wye, PCCS Books.

Casement, P. (1985) *On Learning from the Patient*. London, Tavistock/Routledge.

Casement, P. (1990) *Further Learning from the Patient: The Analytic Space and Process*. London, Tavistock/Routledge.

Cassidy, S. (1987) *Sharing the Darkness: The Spirituality of Caring*. London, DLT.

Clark, S.H. (1990) *Paul Ricoeur*. London, Routledge.

Clarkson, P. (1989) *Gestalt Counselling in Action*. London, Sage.

Clarkson, P. (1992) *Transactional Analysis Psychotherapy: An Integrative Approach.* London, Routledge.

Clarkson, P. (1993) *Fritz Perls.* London, Sage.

Clarkson, P. (1996) 'The Eclectic and Integrative Paradigm' in R. Woolfe and W. Dryden (eds) *Handbook of Counselling Psychology.* London, Sage, pp. 258–83.

Cohn, H.W. (1997) *Existential Thought and Therapeutic Practice.* London, Sage.

Collins, J. and H. Selina (1999) *Introducing Heidegger.* Cambridge, Icon.

Cooper, D.E. (1990) *Existentialism: A Reconstruction.* Oxford, Basil Blackwell.

Cooper, M. (1999) 'If You can't be Jekyll be Hyde: An Existential-Phenomenological Exploration of Lived-Plurality' in J. Rowan and M. Cooper (eds) *The Plural Self.* London, Sage, pp. 51–70.

Cooper, M. (2003) *Existential Therapies.* London, Sage.

Cooper, M. (2005) 'From Self-Objectification to Self-Affirmation: The 'I-Me' and 'I-Self' Relation Stances' in S. Joseph, and R.J. Worsley (eds) *Person-Centred Psychopathology: A Positive Psychology of Mental Health.* Ross-on-Wye, PCCS Books, pp. 60–74.

Cox, M. (1988) *Structuring the Therapeutic Space: Compromise with Chaos.* London, Jessica Kingsley (Revised edition).

Critchley, S. and Bernasconi, R. (eds) (2002) *The Cambridge Companion to Levinas.* Cambridge, UK, Cambridge University Press.

Crossley, N. (1996) *Intersubjectivity: The Fabric of Social Becoming.* London, Sage.

Dainow, S. and C. Bailey (1988) *Developing Skills with People.* Chichester, John Wiley.

Dalal, F. (1998) *Taking the Group Seriously: Towards a Post-Foulkesian Group Analytic Theory.* London, Jessica Kingsley.

Davie, G. (1994) *Religion in Britain since 1945.* Oxford, Blackwell.

Davies, D. and C. Neal (1996) *Pink Therapy.* Milton Keynes, Open University Press.

Dawkins, R. (2006) *The God Delusion.* London, Bantam Books.

Debats, D.L. (1999) 'Sources of Meaning: Significant Commitments in Life' in *Journal of Humanistic Psychology* 39(4), Fall 1999. Thousand Oaks, Sage.

Dryden, W., I. Horton and D. Mearns (1995) *Issues in Professional Counsellor Training.* London, Cassell.

Edelman, G. (1992) *Bright Air, Brilliant Fire: On the Matter of Mind.* London, Allen Lane.

Egan, G. (1990) *The Skilled Helper.* Pacific Grove, California, Brooks Cole (4th edition).

Ellingham, I. (2005) 'Transference Trashed and Transcended'. *Person-Centred Quarterly*, February, 2005.

Elliott, R., J.C. Watson, R.N. Goldman and L.S. Greenberg (2003) *Learning Emotion-Focused Therapy: The Process-Experiential Approach to Change.* Washington, American Psychological Association.

Ellis, W.D. (ed.) (1938) *A Sourcebook of Gestalt Psychology.* London, Kegan Paul, Trench, Trubner and Co.

Eliot, T.S. (1963) *Collected Poems 1909–1962.* London, Faber.

Etherington, K. (2000) *Narrative Approaches to Working with Adult Male Survivors of Child Sexual Abuse: The Clients', the Counsellor's and the Researcher's Story.* London, Jessica Kingsley.

Fairbairn, W.R.D. (1952) *Psychoanalytic Studies of the Personality.* London, Routledge.

Farber, B., D.C. Brink and P.M. Raskin (eds) (1996) *The Psychotherapy of Carl Rogers: Cases and Commentary*. New York, The Guilford Press.

Feltham, C. (1997) 'Challenging the Core Theoretical Model' in *Counselling* 8:2 Rugby, BAC, May 1997.

Frankel, M. and L. Sommerbeck (2007) 'Two Rogers: Congruence and the Change from Client-Centered Therapy to We-Centered Therapy' in *Person-Centered and Experiential Psychotherapies* 6:4, pp. 286–95.

Frankl, V. (1987) *Man's Search for Meaning*. London, Hodder & Stoughton.

Frankland, A. and P. Sanders (1995) *Next Steps in Counselling*. Ross-on-Wye, PCCS Books.

Friedman, M.S. (2002) *Martin Buber: The Life of Dialogue*. London, Routledge (4th edition).

Gardiner, P. (1996) *Kierkegaard*. Oxford, Oxford University Press.

Gendlin, E.T. (1963) 'Subverbal Communication and Therapist Expressivity: Trends in Client-Centered Therapy with Schizophrenics' in *Journal of Existential Psychiatry* 4:14, 105–20.

Gendlin, E.T. (1981) *Focusing*. New York, Bantam Books.

Gendlin, E.T. (1996) *Focusing-Orientated Psychotherapy*. New York, The Guilford Press.

Gendlin, E.T. (1997) *Experiencing and the Creation of Meaning: A Philosophical and Psychological Approach to the Subjective*. Evanston, Northwestern University Press.

Gendlin, E.T., J. Beebe, J. Cassens, M. Klein and R. Oberlander (1968) 'Focusing Ability in Psychotherapy, Personality and Creativity' in J.M. Shlien (ed.) *Research in Psychotherapy* Vol 3, Washington DC, American Psychological Association, pp. 217–41.

Goleman, D. (1996) *Emotional Intelligence*. London, Bloomsbury.

Grant, B. (1990) 'Principled and Instrumental Non-Directiveness in Person-Centered and Client-Centered Therapy'. *Person-Centered Review* 5, pp. 77–88. Reprinted in Cain (2002), pp. 371–7.

Gray, J. (2004) *Consciousness: Creeping Up on the Hard Problem*. Oxford, OUP.

Greenberg, L.S., L.N. Rice and R. Elliott (1993) *Facilitating Emotional Change: The Moment-by-Moment Process*. New York, The Guilford Press.

Guntrip, H. (1971) *Psychology for Ministers and Social Workers*. London, George Allen & Unwin.

Guntrip, H. (1992) *Schizoid Phenomena, Object Relations and the Self*. London, Institute of Psychoanalysis and Karnac Books.

Harris, J.B. (2003) *Gestalt: A New Idiosyncratic Introduction*. Manchester, Gestalt Centre (3rd edition).

Harris, T.A. (2004) *I'm OK – You're OK*. London, Harper Collins.

Hawkins, P. and R. Shohet (1989) *Supervision in the Helping Professions*. Milton Keynes, Open University Press.

Hegel, G.F. (1977) *The Phenomenology of Spirit*. Oxford University Press.

Heidegger, M. (1962) *Being and Time*. Translated by J. Macquarrie and E. Robinson, Oxford, Basil Blackwell.

Heidegger, M. (1995) *The Fundamental Concepts of Metaphysics: World, Finitude, Solitude*. Translated by W. McNeill and N. Walker, Bloomington, University of Indiana Press.

Hermans, H.J.M. and G. Dimaggio (eds) (2004) *The Dialogical Self in Psychotherapy.* Hove, Brunner-Routledge.

Hick, J. (1978) *Evil and the God of Love.* New York, Harper & Row (2nd edition).

Hobson, R.F. (1985) *Forms of Feeling: The Heart of Psychotherapy.* London, Tavistock.

Houston, G. (1990) *The Red Book of Gestalt.* London, The Rochester Foundation (5th edition).

Husserl, E. (1931) *Ideas: General Introduction to Pure Phenomenology.* London, George Allen and Unwin.

Husserl, E. (1973) *Experience and Judgement.* Evanston, Illinois, North Western University Press.

Husserl, E. (1977) *Cartesian Meditation: An Introduction to Metaphysics.* The Hague, Martinus Nijhoff.

Jacobs, M. (1988) *Psychodynamic Counselling in Action.* London, Sage.

Jamison, K.R. (1993) *Touched with Fire: Manic-Depressive Illness and the Artistic Temperament.* New York, Free Press Paperbacks.

Jennings, S. and Å. Minde (1993) *Art Therapy and Dramatherapy: Masks of the Soul.* London, Jessica Kingsley.

Johnson, S.M. (1994) *Character Styles.* New York, W.W. Norton.

Joseph, S. and A. Linley (2006) *Positive Therapy: A Meta-theory for Positive Psychological Practice.* London, Routledge.

Joseph, S. and R.J. Worsley (eds) (2005) *Person-Centred Psychopathology: A Positive Psychology of Mental Health.* Ross-on-Wye, PCCS Books.

Kaufman, W. (ed.) (1956) *Existentialism from Dostoevsky to Sartre.* Cleveland, World Publishing Co.

Kearney, R. (ed.) (1996) *Paul Ricoeur: The Hermeneutics of Action.* London, Sage.

Kierkegaard, S. (1980) *Sickness unto Death.* Translated by H.V. Hong and E.H. Hong, Princeton, Princeton University Press.

Kierkegaard, S. (1985) *Fear and Trembling.* Translated by A. Hannay, Harmondworth, Penguin.

Kirschenbaum, H. and V.L. Henderson (eds) (1990a) *The Carl Rogers Reader.* London, Constable.

Kirschenbaum, H. and V.L. Henderson (eds) (1990b) *Carl Rogers: Dialogues.* London, Constable.

Klein, J. (1987) *Our Need for Others.* London, Routledge.

Klein, M. (1988a) *Love, Guilt and Reparation.* London, Virago.

Klein, M. (1988b) *Envy and Gratiude.* London, Virago.

Knights, B. (1995) *The Listening Reader: Fiction and Poetry for Counsellors and Psychotherapists.* London, Jessica Kingsley.

Kolb, D. (1984) *Experiential Learning.* Englewood Cliffs, NJ, Prentice Hall.

Korb, M., J. Gorrell and V. van der Riet (1989) *Gestalt Therapy: Practice and Theory.* Boston, Allyn & Bacon.

Kuhn, T. (1962) *The Structure of Scientific Revolutions.* Chicago, Chicago University Press.

Lago, C. and M. MacMillan (eds) (1999) *Experiences in Relatedness: Groupwork and the Person-Centred Approach.* Ross-on-Wye, PCCS Books.

Laing, R.D. (1961) *Self and Others.* Harmondsworth, Penguin.

Laing, R.D. and Esterson, A. (1990) *Sanity, Madness and the Family: Families of Schizophrenics*. Harmondsworth, Penguin.

Lake, F. (1986) *Clinical Theology: A Theological and Psychological Basis to Clinical Pastoral Care*. Abridged by M.H. Yeomans, London, Darton Longman and Todd.

Lemma, A. (1996) *Introduction to Psychopathology*. London, Sage.

Levant, R.F. and J.M. Shlien (eds) (1984) *Client-Centered Therapy and the Person-Centered Approach: New Directions in Theory, Research and Practice*. London, Sage.

Levinas, E. (1969) *Totality and Infinity: An Essay on Exteriority*. Translated by A. Lingis, Pittsburgh, Pen., Duquesne University Press.

Levinas, E. (1996) *Basic Philosophical Writings* (edited by A.T. Peperzak, S. Critchley and R. Bernasconi). Bloomington and Indianapolis, Indiana University Press.

Levinas, E. (1998) *Otherwise than Being: Or Beyond Essence*. Translated by A. Lingis, Pittsburgh, Pen., Duquesne University Press.

Levitt, B.E. (ed.) (2008) *Reflections on Human Potential: Bridging the Person-Centred Approach and Positive Psychology*. Ross-on-Wye, PCCS Books.

Lietaer, G. (1998) 'From Non-Directive to Experiential: A Paradigm Unfolding' in Thorne and Lambers (1998), pp. 63–73.

Lietaer, G. (2002) 'The United Colors of Person-Centered and Experiential Psychotherapies' in *Person-Centered and Experiential Psychotherapies* 1:1 and 2, pp. 4–13.

Linley, P.A. and S. Joseph, (eds) (2004) *Positive Psychology in Practice*. Hoboken, N.J., John Wiley and Sons.

Long, E.T. (1968) *Jaspers and Bultmann: A Dialogue Between Philosophy and Theology in the Existentialist Tradition*. North Carolina, Duke University Press.

Luijpen, W.A. (1960) *Existential Phenomenology*. Pittsburgh, Dusquesne University Press.

Lynch, G. (1996) 'Where is the Theology of British Pastoral Counselling?' in *Contact* 121, pp. 22–8.

Lynch, G. (1997a) 'Therapeutic Theory and Social Context: A Social Constructionist Perspective' in *British Journal of Guidance and Counselling* 25:1, pp. 5–15.

Lynch, G. (1997b) 'Words and Silence: Counselling and Psychotherapy after Wittgenstein' in *Counselling* 8:2, Rugby, pp. 126–8.

Lynch, G. (1997c) 'Integrating Christian Faith and the Person-Centred Approach' in *Contact* 124, pp. 10–16.

McLeod, J. (1996) 'The Humanistic Paradigm' in R. Woolfe and W. Dryden (eds) *Handbook of Counselling Psychology*. London, Sage, pp. 133–55.

McLeod, J. (1997) *Narrative and Psychotherapy*. London, Sage.

McNamee, S. and K.J. Gergen (eds) (1992) *Therapy as Social Construction*. London, Sage.

Macquarrie, J. (1966) *Principles of Christian Theology*. London, SCM Press.

Macquarrie, J. (1972/1991) *Existentialism*. Harmondsworth, Pelican/Penguin.

Mahrer, A. (1986) *Therapeutic Experiencing: The Process of Change*. New York, W.W. Norton.

Matthews, E. (1996) *Twentieth-Century French Philosophy*. Oxford University Press.

May, R. (1969) *Love and Will*. New York, W.W. Norton.

May, R. (1982) 'The Problem of Evil: An Open Letter to Carl Rogers' in *Journal of Humanistic Psychology* 22:3, Summer, pp. 10–21, reprinted in Kirschenbaum and Henderson (1990b), pp. 239–51.

Mearns, D. (1994a) *Developing Person-Centred Counselling.* London, Sage.

Mearns, D. (1994b) *The Dance of Psychotherapy* (Videotape of Lecture) University of Sheffield.

Mearns, D. (1996) 'Working at Relational Depth with Clients in Person-Centred Therapy' in *Counselling* 7:6, Rugby BAC November, pp. 306–11.

Mearns, D. (1997) *Person-Centred Counselling Training.* London, Sage.

Mearns, D. (1999) 'Person-Centred Therapy with Configurations of Self' in *Counselling* 10:2, Rugby BAC May, pp. 125–30.

Mearns, D. and Cooper, M. (2005) *Working at Relational Depth in Counselling and Psychotherapy.* London, Sage.

Mearns, D. and B. Thorne (1988/1999/2007) *Person-Centred Counselling in Action.* London, Sage (1st, 2nd and 3rd editions, respectively).

Mearns, D. and B. Thorne (2000) *Person-Centred Therapy Today: New Frontiers in Theory and Practice.* London, Sage.

Mearns, D. and B. Thorne (2007) *Person-Centred Counselling in Action.* London, Sage (3rd edition).

Merleau-Ponty, M. (1962a) *Phenomenology of Perception.* Translated by C. Smith, London, Routledge and Kegan Paul.

Merleau-Ponty, M. (1962b) 'An Unpublished Text' in Merleau-Ponty (1964), chapter one, translated by A.B. Dallery, 'Un inédit de Maurice Merleau-Ponty', *Revue de métaphysique et de morale* 4 Paris (1962) 401–9.

Merleau-Ponty, M. (1964) *The Primacy of Perception.* Translated by J.M. Eadie, Evanston, Northwestern University Press.

Merry, T. (1999) *Learning and Being in Person-Centred Counselling.* Ross-on-Wye, PCCS Books.

Merry, T. (2004) 'Classical Client-Centred Therapy' in P. Sanders (ed.) *The Tribes of the Person-Centred Nation: An Introduction to the Schools of Therapy Related to the Person-Centred Approach.* Ross-on-Wye, PCCS Books, pp. 21–44.

Mitchell, S. (ed.) (1996) *Dramatherapy: Clinical Studies.* London, Jessica Kingsley.

Moncrieff, J. (2008) *The Myth of the Chemical Cure: A Critique of Psychiatric Drug Treatment.* Houndmills, Palgrave.

Moore, J. and C. Purton (eds) (2006) *Spirituality and Counselling: Experiential and Theoretical Perspectives.* Ross-on-Wye, PCCS Books.

Moustakas, C. (1994) *Phenomenological Research Methods.* London, Sage.

O'Connor, F. (1963) *My Oedipus Complex and Other Stories.* Harmondsworth, Penguin.

O'Donohue, J. (1997) *Anam Cara: Spiritual Wisdom from the Celtic World.* London, Bantam Press.

Ogden, T.H. (1992) *The Matrix of the Mind: Object Relations and the Psychoanalytic Dialogue.* London, Karnac.

O'Leary, C. (1999) *Counselling Couples and Families: A Person-Centred Approach.* London, Sage.

Parkin, D. (ed.) (1985) *The Anthropology of Evil.* Oxford, Basil Blackwell.

Patterson, C.H. (2000) *Understanding Psychotherapy: Fifty Years of Client-Centred Theory and Practice.* Ross-on-Wye, PCCS Books.

Pattison, G. (1999) *Anxious Angels: A Retrospective View of Religious Existentialism.* London, Macmillan.

Payne, M. (2006) *Narrative Therapy.* London, Sage.

Perls, F.S. (1992) *Gestalt Therapy Verbatim*. Gouldsboro, ME, Gestalt Journal Press.

Perls, F.S., R.F. Hefferline and P. Goodman (1973) *Gestalt Therapy: Excitement and Growth in the Human Personality*. Harmondsworth, Penguin.

Polt, R. (1999) *Heidegger: An Introduction*. London, UCL Press.

Poole, R. and H. Stangerup (eds) (1989) *A Kierkegaard Reader: Texts and Narratives*. London, Fourth Estate.

Prouty, G.F. (1990) 'Pre–Therapy: a Theoretical Evolution in the Person-Centered/Experiential Psychotherapy of Schizophrenia and Retardation' in G. Lietaer, J. Rombauts and R. Van Balen (eds) *Client-Centered and Experiential Psychotherapy in the Nineties*. Leuven, Leuven University Press, pp. 645–58.

Prouty, G.F. (1994) *Theoretical Evolutions in Person-Centered/Experiential Therapy: Applications to Schizophrenic and Retarded Psychoses*. Westport, CT Praeger.

Prouty, G.F. (2007) 'The Hallucination as the Unconscious Self' in R.J. Worsley and S. Joseph (eds) *Person-Centred Practice: Case Studies in Positive Psychology*. Ross-on-Wye, PCCS Books, pp. 169–83.

Prouty, G.F., D. Van Werde and M. Pörtner (2002) *Pre-therapy: Reaching Contact-Impaired Clients*. Ross-on-Wye, PCCS Books.

Purton, C. (1998) 'Unconditional Positive Regard and Its Spiritual Implications' in Thorne and Lambers pp. 23–37.

Purton, C. (2007) *The Focus-Orientated Counselling Primer*. Ross-on-Wye, PCCS Books.

Read, J. (2004) 'The Invention of "Schizophrenia"' in J. Read, L.R. Mosher and R. Bentall (eds) *Models of Madness: Psychological, Social and Biological Approaches to Schizophrenia*. London, Brunner-Routledge, pp. 21–34.

Read, J., L.R. Mosher and R. Bentall (eds) (2004) *Models of Madness: Psychological, Social and Biological Approaches to Schizophrenia*. London, Brunner-Routledge.

Rennie, D. (1998) *Person-Centred Counselling: An Experiential Approach*. London, Sage.

Rennie, D. (2006) 'Radical Reflexivity: Rationale for an Experiential Person-Centered Approach to Counselling and Psychotherapy' in *Person-Centered and Experiential Psychotherapies* 5:2, pp. 114–26.

Rice, L.N. (1974) 'The Evocative Function of the Therapist' in D. Wexler and L.N. Rice (eds) *Innovations in Client-Centred Therapy*. New York, Wiley.

Rice, L.N. (1984) 'Client tasks in Client-centered Therapy' in R.F. Levant and J.M. Shlien (eds) *Client-centered Therapy and the Person-centered Approach*. New York, Praeger, pp. 182–202.

Ricoeur, P. (1975) *The Rule of Metaphor*. London, Routledge & Kegan Paul.

Rilke, R. (1952) *Duino Elegies*. London, Hogarth Press.

Rogers, C. (1951) *Client-Centred Therapy*. London, Constable.

Rogers, C. and R. Dymond (1954) *Psychotherapy and Personality Change*. Chicago, University of Chicago.

Rogers, C. (1957a) 'The Necessary and Sufficient Conditions of Therapeutic Personality Change' in *Journal of Consulting Psychology* 21, pp. 95–103.

Rogers, C. (1957b) 'A Therapist's View of the Good Life: The Fully Functioning Person' in Rogers (1967) pp. 184–96.

Rogers, C. (1957c) 'A Process Conception of Psychotherapy' in Rogers (1967) pp. 125–59.

Rogers, C. (1959) 'A Theory of Therapy, Personality and Interpersonal Relationships, As Developed in the Client-Centered Framework' in S. Koch (ed.) *Psychology, A Study of Science: 3. Formulations of the Person and the Social Context.* New York, McGraw-Hill, pp. 184–256.

Rogers, C. (1963) 'The Actualizing Tendency in Relation to "Motives" and to Consciousness' in M.R. Jones (ed.) *Nebraska Symposium on Motivation.* Lincoln, University of Nebraska Press, pp. 1–24.

Rogers, C. (1967) *On Becoming a Person.* London, Constable.

Rogers, C. (1970) *On Encounter Groups.* New York, Harper & Row.

Rogers, C. (1977) *Three Approaches to Psychotherapy II, Part 1 – Carl Rogers (Client Centered Therapy).* Corona del Mar, CA, Psychological and Educational Films.

Rogers, C. (1978) *Carl Rogers on Personal Power.* London, Constable.

Rogers, C. (1980) *A Way of Being.* Boston, Houghton Mifflin.

Rogers, C. (1982) 'Reply to Rollo May's Letter' in *Journal of Humanistic Psychology* 22:4, Fall 85–9, reprinted in Kirschenbaum and Henderson (1990b) 251–5.

Rogers, C. (1986a) 'A Client-Centered/Person-Centered Approach to Therapy' in I. Kutash and A. Wolf (eds) (1986) *Psychotherapist's Casebook.* San Francisco, Jossey-Bass, pp. 197–208.

Rogers, C. (1986b) 'Reflection of Feeling' in *Person-Centered Review* 1:4, pp. 375–7.

Rogers, C. (1987) 'Transference' in *Person-Centered Review* 2:2 May, London, Sage, pp. 182–8.

Rogers, C. and B. Stevens (1973) *Person to Person.* London, Souvenir Press.

Rowan, J. (1990) *Subpersonalities: The People Inside Us.* London, Routledge.

Sachse, R. (2006) 'From Client-Centred to Clarification-Oriented Psychotherapy' in *PCEP*, 3:1, pp. 19–35.

Sanders, P. (2000) 'Mapping Person-Centred Approaches to Counselling and Psychotherapy' in *Person Centred Practice* 8:2, pp. 62–74.

Sanders, P. (ed.) (2004) *Tribes of the Person-Centred Nation: An Introduction to the Schools of Therapy Related to the Person-Centred Approach.* Ross-on-Wye: PCCS Books.

Sanders, P. (2005) 'Principled and Strategic Opposition to the Medicalisation of Distress and All Its Apparatus' in S. Joseph and R.J. Worsley (eds) *Person-Centred Psychopathology: A Positive Psychology of Mental Health.* Ross-on-Wye, PCCS Books, pp. 21–42.

Sanders, P. (2006) *The Person-Centred Counselling Primer.* Ross-on-Wye, PCCS Books.

Sanders, P. (2007a) 'In Place of the Medical Model: Person-Centred Alternatives to the Medicalisation of Distress' in R.J. Worsley and S. Joseph (eds) (2007) *Person-Centred Practice: Case Studies in Positive Psychology.* Ross-on-Wye, PCCS Books, pp.184–199.

Sanders, P. (ed.) (2007b) *The Contact Work Primer: A Concise, Accessible and Comprehensive Introduction to Pre-Therapy and the Work of Garry Prouty.* Ross-on-Wye, PCCS Books.

Sartre, J.-P. (1996) *L'existentialisme est un humanisme.* Paris, Editions Gallimard.

Schmid, P.F. (1998) '"Face to Face" – The Art of Encounter' in B. Thorne and E. Lambers (eds), pp. 74–90.

Schmid, P.F. (2006) '"In the Beginning There is Community". Implications and Challenges of the Belief in a Triune God and a Person-Centered Approach' in J. Moore & C. Purton (Eds). *Spirituality and Counselling: Experiential and Theoretical Perspectives* (pp. 227–46). Ross-on-Wye: PCCS Books.

Schön, D.A. (1987) *Educating the Reflective Practitioner.* San Francisco, Jossey-Bass.

Searles, H. (1961) 'Schizophrenia and the Inevitability of Death' in *Psychiatric Quarterly* 35, pp. 631–55.

Segal, J. (1992) *Melanie Klein.* London, Sage.

Shaffer, J. (1978) *Humanistic Psychology.* Englewood Cliffs, Prentice-Hall.

Shakespeare, W. (1951) *Henry V* in *William Shakespeare: The Complete Works*, in P. Alexander (ed.), London, Collins.

Shakespeare, W. (1964) *The Sonnets*, in W. Burto (ed.), New York, Signet.

Shlien, J.M. (2000) Personal correspondence between John Shlien and Pete Sanders referred to in Sanders (2000), p. 67.

Shlien, J.M. (2003) *To Lead an Honorable Life: Invitations to Think about Client-Centered Therapy and the Person-Centered Approach*, P. Sanders (ed.). Ross-on-Wye, PCCS Books.

Sills, C., S. Fish and P. Lapworth (1995) *Gestalt Counselling.* Bicester, Winslow Press.

Silverstone, L. (1994) 'Art Therapy the Person-Centred Way: Its Relevance in Counselling' in *Counselling* 5:6, Rugby BAC, November, pp. 291–3.

Silverstone, L. (1997) *Art Therapy the Person-Centred Way: Art and the Development of the Person.* London, Jessica Kingsley.

Sinclair, A. (1989) 'Concepts of Tragedy in Unamuno and Kierkegaard' in N. Round (ed.) *Re-reading Unamuno.* Glasgow Colloquium Papers 1: University of Glasgow, Department of Hispanic Studies.

Slife, B.D., C. Hope and R.S. Nebeker (1999) 'Examining the Relationship between Religious Spirituality and Psychological Science' in *Journal of Humanistic Psychology* 39:2, London, Sage.

Sperry, R.W. (1995) 'Consciousness' in *Journal of Humanistic Psychology* 35:2, Spring, Thousand Oaks, pp. 7–33.

Spinelli, E. (1989/2005) *The Interpreted World: Introduction to Phenomenological Psychology.* London, Sage.

Spinelli, I. (2007) Practising Existential Psychotherapy: The Relational World. London, Sage.

Sommerbeck, E. (2005) 'The Complementarity between Client-Centred Therapy and Psychiatry: The Theory and the Practice' in S. Joseph, and R.J. Worsley (eds) *Person-Centred Psychopathology: A Positive Psychology of Mental Health.* Ross-on-Wye, PCCS Books, pp. 110–127.

Standal, S. (1954) *The Need for Positive Regard. A Contribution to Client-Centered Theory.* Unpublished PhD. thesis, University of Chicago.

Stephens, J.O. (1989) *Awareness.* London, Eden Grove.

Stewart, I. and V. Joines (1987) *T.A. Today.* Nottingham, Lifespace.

Stewart, I. (1989) *Transactional Analysis Counselling in Action.* London, Sage.

Stewart, I. (1996) *Developing Transactional Analysis Counselling.* London, Sage.

Strasser, F. and A. Strasser (1997) *Existential Time-Limited Therapy: The Wheel of Existence.* Chichester, John Wiley.

Sugarman, L. (1986) *Life-Span Development: Concepts, Theories and Interventions.* London, Routledge.

Surin, K. (1986) *Theology and the Problem of Evil.* Oxford, Basil Blackwell.

Thorne, B. (1991) *Person-Centred Counselling: Therapeutic and Spiritual Dimensions.* London, Whurr.

Thorne, B. (1992) *Carl Rogers.* London, Sage.

Thorne, B. (1998) *Person-Centred Counselling and Christian Spirituality.* London, Whurr.

Thorne, B. (2002) *The Mystical Power of Person-Centred Therapy: Hope beyond Despair.* London, Whurr.

Thorne, B. and E. Lambers (eds) (1998) *Person-Centred Therapy: A European Perspective.* London, Sage.

Tillich, P. (1952) *The Courage to Be.* New Haven, Yale University Press.

Tisdale, J.R. (1994) 'Transpersonal Psychology and Jesus' in *Journal of Humanistic Psychology* 34:3, Summer, Thousand Oaks, pp. 31–47.

Toukmanian, S.G. (1992) 'Studying the Client's Processes and their Outcome in Psychotherapy' in S.G. Toukmanian and D.L. Rennie (eds) *Psychotherapy Process Research: Paradigmatic and Narrative Approaches.* London, Sage.

Trivasse, K. (2004) *Walking Towards the Mosque. Contact,* Pastoral Monograph No. 13.

Tudor, K. (2000) 'The Case of the Lost Conditions' in *Counselling* 11:1, Rugby BAC, February, pp. 33–7.

Tudor, K. and Worrall, M. (eds) (2004) *Freedom to Practice: Person-Centred Approaches to Supervision.* Ross-on-Wye, PCCS Books.

Unamuno, M. de (1977) *The Tragic Sense of Life.* Translated by A. Kerrigan, Princeton University Press.

Vanaerschot, G. (1993) 'Empathy as Releasing Several Microprocesses in the Client' in Brazier (1993).

Van Deurzen-Smith, E. (1995) 'Letting the Client's Life Touch Yours' in *Changes: An International Journal of Psychology and Psychotherapy* 13:4, Chichester and New York, John Wiley & Sons.

Van Deurzen-Smith, E. (1997) *Everyday Mysteries, Existential Dimensions of Psychotherapy.* Hove, Brunner-Routledge.

Van Werde, D. (2002) 'A Contact Milieu' in G.F. Prouty, D. Van Werde and M. Pörtner (eds) *Pre-therapy: Reaching Contact-impaired Clients.* Ross-on-Wye, PCCS Books, pp. 77–114.

Van Werde, D. (2005) 'Facing Psychotic Functioning: Person-Centred Contact Work in Residential Psychiatric Care' in S. Joseph and R.J. Worsley (eds) *Person-Centred Psychopathology: A Positive Psychology of Mental Health.* Ross-on-Wye, PCCS Books, pp. 158–68.

Van Werde, D. (2007) The Falling Man: Pre-therapy Applied to Somatic Hallucinating' in R.J. Worsley and S. Joseph (eds) Person-*Centred Practice: Case Studies in Positive Psychology.* Ross-on-Wye, PCCS Books, pp. 135–41.

Villas-Boas Bowen, M. (1996) 'The Myth of Nondirectiveness' in Farber *et al.* (1996) pp. 84–94.

Warner, M. (2002) 'Luke's Dilemmas: A Client-Centered/Experiential Model of Processing with a Schizophrenic Thought Disorder' in J.C. Watson, R.N. Goldman and M.S. Warner (eds) *Client-Centered and Experiential Psychotherapy in the 21st Century: Advances in Theory, Research and Practice.* Ross-on-Wye, PCCS Books, pp. 459–72.

Warner, M. (2007) 'Luke's Process: A Positive View of Schizophrenic Thought Disorder' in R.J. Worsley, and S. Joseph (eds) *Person-Centred Practice: Case Studies in Positive Psychology*. Ross-on-Wye, PCCS Books, pp. 142–55.

Weishaar, M.E. (1993) *Aaron T. Beck*. London, Sage.

Wertz, F.J. (1998) 'The Humanistic Movement in Psychology' in *Journal of Humanistic Psychology* 38:1, Winter, Thousand Oaks, pp. 42–70.

West, W. (2000) *Psychotherapy and Spirituality*. London, Sage.

Wilkins, P. (1997) 'Congruence and Countertransference' in *Counselling* 8:1, February, pp. 36–41.

Winter, D. (1996) 'The Constructivist Paradigm' in R. Woolfe and W. Dryden (eds) (1996) *Handbook of Counselling Psychology*. London, Sage, pp. 219–39.

Wiseman, H. (1998) 'Training Counsellors in the Process-Experiential Approach' in *British Journal of Guidance and Counselling* 26:1, January, pp. 105–18.

Wittgenstein, L. (1963) *Philosophical Investigations*. Oxford, Blackwell.

Worsley, R.J. (1993) 'Bright Air, Brilliant Fire' in *Theology* No. 773 September/ October, pp. 395–6.

Worsley, R.J. (1996) *Human Freedom and the Logic of Evil*. London, Macmillan.

Worsley, R.J. (1997) 'Absolute or Metaphor: Theological Critiques of Pastoral Counselling' in *Contact* 124, pp. 17–23.

Worsley, R.J. (2000a) 'Can we Talk about the Spirituality of Counselling?' in *Counselling* 11:2, Rugby BAC, March, pp. 89–91.

Worsley, R.J. (2000b) 'Psychotherapy and Spirituality' in *Counselling* 11:4, Rugby BAC, May, p. 218.

Worsley, R.J. (2000c) 'Affirming Spirituality' in *The Newsletter of the Association of Pastoral and Spiritual Care and Counselling*. November, pp. 8–10.

Worsley, R.J. (2001) 'Problems with Evil' in *Person-Centred Practice* 9:1.

Worsley, R.J. (2004) 'Integrating with Integrity' in P. Sanders (ed.) *Tribes of the Person-Centred Nation: An Introduction to the Schools of Therapy Related to the Person-Centred Approach*. Ross-on-Wye: PCCS Books.

Worsley, R. (2006) 'Emmanuel Levinas: Resource and challenge for therapy'. *Person-Centered and Experiential Psychotherapies* 5:3, pp. 208–20.

Worsley, R.J. (2007a) *The Integrative Counselling Primer*. Ross-on-Wye, PCCS Books.

Worsley, R.J. (2007b) 'Diagnosis, Stuckness and Encounter: Existential Meaning in Long-Term Depression' in Worsley, R.J. and S. Joseph (eds) *Person-Centred Practice: Case Studies in Positive Psychology*. Ross-on-Wye, PCCS Books, pp. 98–114.

Worsley, R.J. (2008a) 'Lived Experience'. *Therapy Today* 19:1, Rugby, BACP, pp. 14–17.

Worsley, R.J. (2008b) 'More than Meets the Eye.' *Therapy Today* 19:2 , Rugby, BACP, pp. 34–36.

Worsley, R.J. and S. Joseph (eds) (2007) *Person-Centred Practice: Case Studies in Positive Psychology*. Ross-on-Wye, PCCS Books.

Wyatt, G. and P. Sanders (2002) *Contact and Perception*. Ross-on-Wye, PCCS Books.

Yalom, I.D. (1980) *Existential Psychotherapy*. New York, Basic Books.

Yalom, I.D. (1989) *Love's Executioner and Other Tales of Psychotherapy*. Harmondsworth, Penguin.

Yalom, I.D. (1995) *The Theory and Practice of Group Psychotherapy*. New York, Basic Books.

Yalom, I.D. (2002) *The Gift of Therapy: Reflections on Being a Therapist*. London, Piatkus.

Zinker, J. (1978) *Creative Process in Gestalt Therapy*. New York, Random House.

# Index

Note: Case studies are listed below in *italics*

9 780230 213159